A Companion Volume to Dr. Jay A. Goldstein's *Betrayal by the Brain*

A Guide for Patients and Their Physicians

The Haworth Library of the
Medical Neurobiology of Somatic Disorders
Neuroimmunoendocrine Networks
in Health & Illness

Volume I: *Chronic Fatigue Syndromes: The Limbic Hypothesis*

Volume II: *Betrayal by the Brain: The Neurologic Basis of Chronic Fatigue Syndrome, Fibromyalgia Syndrome, and Related Neural Network Disorders*

Editor-in-Chief

Jay A. Goldstein, MD, Director
Chronic Fatigue Syndrome Institute, Anaheim, California

A Companion Volume to Dr. Jay A. Goldstein's *Betrayal by the Brain*

A Guide for Patients and Their Physicians

Katie Courmel

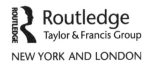

Routledge
Taylor & Francis Group

NEW YORK AND LONDON

Published by

The Haworth Medical Press, an imprint of The Haworth Press, Inc., 10 Alice Street, Binghamton, NY 13904-1580

Transferred to Digital Printing 2011 by Routledge
711 Third Avenue, New York, NY 10017
2 Park Square, Milton Park, Abingdon, Oxon, OX14 4RN

DISCLAIMER
Medicine is an ever-changing science. As new research and clinical experience broaden our knowledge, changes in treatment and drug therapy are required. While many suggestions for drug usages are made herein, the book is intended for educational purposes only, and the author, editor, and publisher do not accept liability in the event of negative consequences incurred as a result of information presented in this book. We do not claim that this information is necessarily accurate by the rigid, scientific standard applied for medical proof, and therefore make no warranty, expressed or implied, with respect to the material herein contained. Therefore the patient is urged to consult his or her own physician prior to following a course of treatment. The physician is urged to check the product information sheet included in the package of each drug he or she plans to administer to be certain the protocol followed is not in conflict with the manufacturer's inserts. When a discrepancy arises between these inserts and information in this book, the physician is encouraged to use his or her best professional judgement.

Cover designed by Marylouise Doyle.

ISBN 0-7890-0119-5

A Companion Volume to Dr. Jay A. Goldstein's *Betrayal by the Brain:* A Guide for Patients and Their Physicians

Library of Congress Cataloging-in-Publication Data

Goldstein, Jay A.
    Betrayal by the brain : the neurologic basis of chronic fatigue syndrome, fibromyalgia syndrome, and related neural network disorders / Jay A. Goldstein.
        p.   cm.
    Companion v. to: Chronic fatigue syndromes : the limbic hypothesis / Jay A. Goldstein. ©1993.
    Includes bibliographical references and index.
    ISBN 1-56024-977-3 (alk. paper).
    1. Chronic fatigue syndrome. 2. Fibromyalgia. 3. Psychoneuroimmunology. 4. Neural networks (Neurobiology). 5. Limbic system. I. Goldstein, Jay A. Chronic fatigue syndromes. II. Title.
    [DNLM: 1. Nervous System Diseases. 2. Nerve Net–physiopathology. 3. Fatigue Syndrome, Chronic–physiopathology. 4. Fatigue Syndrome, Chronic–drug therapy. 5. Fibromyalgia–physiopathology. 6. Fibromyalgia–drug therapy. WL 300 G624b 1994]
RB 150.F37G649 1994
616.8'4–dc20
DNLM/DLC
for Library of Congress   95-51124
                                                                                                                                        CIP

Publisher's Note
The publisher has gone to great lengths to ensure the quality of this reprint but points out that some imperfections in the original may be apparent.

CONTENTS

ABOUT THE AUTHOR

Katie Courmel was a software development manager until 1992, when she became disabled by a pelvic injury that developed into fibromyalgia and chronic fatigue syndrome. Fortunately, she was diagnosed within one year of acquiring symptoms, and has, since that time, done extensive research on both diseases. Ms. Courmel encourages other CFS/FMS patients to learn to be their own "patient advocates," having found through personal experience that most physicians do not establish long-term care relationships with this patient group unless the patients aggressively pursue such treatment.

After becoming disabled, Ms. Courmel attempted to enrich her life by exploring the reaches of her creative right brain. She subsequently learned the art of stained glass and received a number of awards before losing the use of her hands. Once an avid mountain climber and a long-distance European trekker, Ms. Courmel still enjoys short hikes in the Colorado mountains and Utah deserts with her husband and four dogs. Finding creative distractions from the pain and respecting your body's limits are the essentials, she believes, for living life to the fullest. "When you focus on the disease, you give it power over your life," she cautions. "Look for the gift that lies behind every difficult situation."

Introduction

I am a former software development project manager for a large computer firm. I am on disability from that occupation as a result of a 1992 injury to my sacral ligaments and sacroiliac joints caused by a yoga maneuver I obviously wasn't ready for–the plow. If you are not familiar with the move, it involves lying on your back and stretching your legs so your toes hang over your head and then staying there for about ten minutes. In retrospect, however, I believe I *was* ready for what the injury brought me. Earlier that day, a major implementation had received its long-awaited go-ahead. That evening, I entered my beginning yoga class with an intent to wind down and relax. Well, I got plenty of time to relax over the next four years (to date); the pain was a side effect I had not intended. I often admired my body for holding together when the going was tough and letting go only when given permission. Usually "letting go" just meant getting a cold, having a week of rest, and getting on with things. This time, my body meant to have a much longer break.

Somewhere in the ensuing years of physical therapy, acupuncture, chiropractic treatment, and massage, in an attempt to stabilize my joints and reverse the compensatory scoliosis I developed fibromyalgia. Of course, I took the blame at first. I had no reason to be hurting in "those" places . . . I must not be doing my exercises right. Then, in an attempt to broaden my homebound existence, I traveled to a Bluegrass Festival in Telluride, Colorado, where I picked up a nasty virus. Most of the viral symptoms went away after two or three weeks, but a chronic low-grade fever remained. Thus, chronic fatigue syndrome (CFS) entered my life.

I went through the natural grieving that is a part of any loss, and I tried valiantly to redefine my life. I tried baking desserts for a gourmet restaurant for a while, but I had to give that up because it was too demanding and fatiguing. Then, I became an award-winning stained-glass artist, until fibromyalgia took away the use of my hands for that type of work. Finally, I struggled to the realization that I am not what I do, that I am of value because of who I am. "We need to remember that we are human beings," not "human doings," as someone has said.

Through the years, I have spent countless dollars and have tried everything from naturopathy to crystals to flower essences–all to no avail. I alternated between Western medicine and holistic medicine, becoming frustrated with one and seeking out the other.

I met Dr. Goldstein through an interesting turn of events. Sometime after I developed CFS, I began to experience a type of seizure that occurred when I was falling asleep or felt chilled. Early on, I would have as many as fifty of them in a day. They were very unnerving and caused a great deal of pain since my entire body would jerk uncontrollably. Neurologists said it was psychosomatic, as did the Mayo Clinic. So, I started a letter-writing campaign to FMS/CFS researchers to see if anyone had encountered it. After reading an article in *Fibromyalgia Network* about Dr. Goldstein's work and its connection with the autonomic nervous system, I decided that if anyone could figure this out, he could. Dr. Goldstein was the only doctor to respond to my letter of pleading and despair. He had seen my symptom–pseudo-seizures–in CFS patients and believed he could help. We then discussed his treatment protocol, and since I was preparing for sacroiliac joint fusion surgery, he suggested I try the protocol to relieve my CFS/FMS symptoms before undertaking such a major surgery.

So, in September 1995, I traveled to California for a week with Dr. Goldstein. I remember going with a great deal of blind faith, as I knew almost nothing about the protocol, except that it had to do with drugs–many of them. I had always been wary of drugs because of my hypersensitivity. I always experienced their "uncommon" side effects. Although 95 percent of Dr. Goldstein's patients obtain relief from his protocol, relief was not to occur for me that week in September 1995. The week is still something of a blur to me, filled with heavy emotional undertones of hope and disappointment. Dr. Goldstein has not given up on me, so I have not given up either. He continues to work in cooperation with my primary care physician to try new drugs to find the one that works for me.

While in California, I picked up a copy of Dr. Goldstein's book, *Betrayal by the Brain*, and sat down for a thorough reading. I was able to grasp the Introduction—beyond that, he lost me. I have a BS in Biology and a minor in Chemistry, so it is reasonable to assume I might have an advantage over the average person, but not so. I decided then and there that Dr. Goldstein's work was too valuable to be so inaccessible because of its complexity to the people who crave an understanding of it the most—those who suffer with CFS and FMS. So, I decided to create this companion volume for my fellow patients, written in common terminology, and simplified as much as possible without sacrificing the body of information that one must understand to appreciate the complexity of these disorders. I am hoping that this book will help you approach Dr. Goldstein's protocol with an open mind and make the decision to try it for yourself. I am also hoping that when you go, my experiences and insights with the treatment itself will prepare you for what is coming so you will feel at ease and can maintain an even emotional keel. Miracles are happening in the lives of CFS and FMS patients every day—thanks to Dr. Goldstein. One of these miracles could be yours, and someday, one of them will be mine.

May God bless you in your search for health and bless Dr. Goldstein for having the compassion to dedicate his career to helping us, in the face of disbelief, derision, and mockery from many of his fellow physicians. The day will come when his work gains the respect it deserves. "A prophet hath no honor in his own country" (John 4:44).

Dr. Jay Goldstein's Drug Treatment Protocol

If you are about to receive Dr. Goldstein's treatment protocol for FMS or CFS, either in Dr. Goldstein's office or under the administration of your local physician, prepare yourself for a unique, unusual, sometimes scary, often perplexing, and hopefully miraculous, "leap of faith" experience. This guide will help you deal with the uneasiness you may be feeling. Hopefully it will also help you understand, in everyday language, what the protocol can accomplish and how it can be so successful.

Most patients check in at their doctor's office, wait until the doctor has finished with the previous patient(s), spend 10 to 15 minutes with the doctor, and leave with a prescription and instructions to "keep in touch."

With Dr. Goldstein, you may stay in the office for one day or as much as a week if you are an out-of-state patient. You will receive drugs throughout the day, some days as many as seven to eight different drugs. These drugs work together with very little interaction. For this reason, you can safely take them in rapid succession. Also, they cause few adverse effects and their onset of action is usually rapid, within 30 to 60 minutes. Although the treatment protocol lists 23 standard drugs, Dr. Goldstein will individually tailor your treatment plan, based on your medical history, past drug experience, and your reactions to drugs you encounter as you progress through the protocol.

The ultimate goal of the treatment protocol is to find the drug or combination of drugs that return you to "normal." This means that your pain disappears, you feel revitalized, your head feels clear, and your mental acuity and memory improves. Obviously, the extent of the response will vary with your initial symptoms and their severity. As you progress through the protocol, you are watching and waiting for changes like these to occur.

Dr. Goldstein's success rate with this protocol is very impressive and is improving along with the growth in his clinical practice. About 50 percent of new patients feel dramatically improved after the first day; 25 percent more are better on the second; 20 percent more eventually respond to treatment, leaving 5 percent whom Dr. Goldstein is unable to help very much.

Dr. Goldstein's philosophy is to make treatments as cost-effective for the patient as possible while not sacrificing safety and efficacy. He has devised inexpensive therapies to replace more costly ones. His vast reservoir of patient history allows him to forego many expensive medical tests because he can reliably predict their outcomes.

HOW SAFE IS THIS PROTOCOL?

Dr. Goldstein has now received funding to perform a double-blind, placebo-controlled study of his protocol. While many physicians consider offering this protocol prior to this study to be unethical, Dr. Goldstein believes it is unethical to withhold treatment if the benefit to the patient outweighs the risk.

Dr. Goldstein's treatment uses FDA-approved medications for off-label indications. An off-label indication refers to a drug approved for one use and found to be effective (but not officially approved) for another condition. Forty percent of drugs prescribed are off-label indications.

SHOULD I GO ALONE OR TAKE A COMPANION?

The answer to this question will depend on a number of factors, including how far you must travel to reach Dr. Goldstein, the severity of your symptoms, your general sensitivity to medication, and your feelings about what you are about to go through. I can offer you my personal advice, since I came alone from out-of-state. I can also offer my observations about those accompanied in their journey from both near and far.

Generally, I would advise that you bring someone with you–preferably someone healthy! I stayed in the treatment program for five days. For four out of those five days, I would have felt unsafe driving a car because I felt drunk, light-headed, and generally "out of it." (I chose to walk each day to and from the clinic and the nearby hotel.) But I am also excessively sensitive to drugs—so take that into consideration.

From an emotional standpoint, if your spouse, your significant other, or a friend can be there for you, their presence can only help. You may find yourself experiencing drastic mood swings—more than you normally do. This can result from drugs that affect the emotion center of the brain or from the disappointment you may feel if one drug after another does not work and you pass yet another day without success. Although you will be happy for those around you who are helped, it is a bittersweet happiness if you are still suffering.

WHAT TO EXPECT DURING YOUR
INITIAL CONSULTATION

If you visit Dr. Goldstein's office, you may spend as much as two or three hours of your first day in an initial consultation with the doctor. This involves a detailed reading of your entire case history, with questions and answers interjected. During this period, Dr. Goldstein will begin his drug treatment protocol, starting with those drugs that have the most fast-acting profile. He may try *naphazoline HCl* eye drops, which may take effect within seconds. He may also try *nitroglycerine* under your tongue, which may act within minutes. You will then take a series of tablets or capsules that are longer- acting, taking effect within 30 to 45 minutes.

Throughout this process, Dr. Goldstein will frequently ask how you are feeling. If you suffer from pain, he will check the sensitivity of a few select FMS "tender points" to help assess the effectiveness of a drug. If you suffer primarily from fatigue and find a drug that revives you, Dr. Goldstein may have you run up and down stairs to see if the drug really works. If cognitive disorders are a main complaint, you might read and discuss a magazine article after the administration of a drug that makes your head feel clearer.

If he believes it will be helpful, Dr. Goldstein may refer you for neuropsychological testing to assess your level of cognitive impairment, if that is a significant part of your symptomology. He may, on rare occasions, refer you for a brain SPECT (single photon emission computerized tomography) scan, which will give him a graphic readout of blood flow within your brain. This is usually unnecessary, as Dr. Goldstein has seen very consistent results over the years in his patient population and chooses not to ask patients to incur the additional expense of these tests. However, if you need medical evidence for a disability claim or lawsuit, Dr. Goldstein can make arrangements for you to receive these tests in the local area.

THE WAITING ROOM

At the conclusion of your initial consultation, you will then take a seat in the waiting room along with the other patients who are being treated that day. Many of them will be following the same ordered drug protocol that you have now embarked upon. It can be comforting to compare any side effects you may be feeling with a particular drug and to talk to patients who are farther along in the protocol about what is to come.

Dr. Goldstein will check in with all the patients in the waiting room at 15 to 30-minute intervals. He will ask whether a drug has made you feel better or worse and ask you to describe your sensations. Once enough time has passed for the drug to have exerted its effect, you will take another. In addition to tablets and capsules, you may also receive injected medications as the protocol progresses and, if necessary, an intravenous (IV) drip of *lidocaine.*

If you have had positive results with a drug on a previous day, it is not unusual for Dr. Goldstein to try that drug again on a subsequent day. This is because it may have worked in conjunction with the drug administered just before or after it, rather than effecting your symptoms singly. This kind of testing allows Dr. Goldstein to develop a multi-drug treatment program.

The most exciting patients to interact with are those who are returning for treatments that have proven successful. Their before- and -after stories will give you hope and build your trust in the process.

You will also meet some of the five percent of patients that are Dr. Goldstein's greatest challenges because they seem to resist all treatment efforts. Their courage will be obvious, but so may be their depression. Be careful to maintain your own center and not be discouraged too much. You will need your strength–physically, mentally, and emotionally–in the days to come. Get outside if you can; take in some fresh air and walk for a little while when you feel drained from taking on too much of the burden of those who are suffering. You will realize very quickly that the waiting room becomes a support group whose dynamics change daily with the influx of new patients. The support group can become a "wailing wall" on some days–so just be aware of your own whining threshold!

Each day you are also likely to witness an "epiphany" or two, that magical moment when someone discovers a drug in the protocol that produces relief. The impact is very profound for all sharing the experience. The healing is visceral and palpable. You would swear from their eyes that they had seen the face of God. Tension will melt from their faces and their bodies, and they will rediscover the joy of movement often denied them for years. Dancing is quite common!

THE EFFECTS OF SO MANY DRUGS

Dr. Goldstein refers to his protocol as an "immersion" process, so it is not unusual for patients to feel that they are receiving an onslaught of drugs–given their previous expectations and warnings from physicians about drug interactions. Also, many patients with such chronic diseases as FMS or CFS try to limit their drug intake to reach a point of balance between presence of mind and bodily comfort. During treatment, your body may also validate this concern, with the effects of the drugs seeming to overlap to the point that you can't discern which drug is causing what effect. For this reason, Dr. Goldstein is very diligent in monitoring how all patients are feeling every 15 to 30 minutes. If you should begin to experience any adverse reactions, Dr. Goldstein often has a drug that will reverse the effects of the drug causing your discomfort. Reactions can run the gamut from feeling "out of it," sedated, anxious, or nauseous, to experiencing tingling sensations. You may also experience a partial amelioration of your symptoms. For example, your joints may begin to feel better while your fatigue or "tender point" pain remains unchanged.

As your treatment day progresses, Dr. Goldstein will assess your ability to tolerate additional drugs based on your response to previous drugs and the duration of effect of those drugs. Generally, your day will run from 10 a.m. until 3 or 4 p.m., but if you feel overwhelmed by the effects of the drugs, just tell Dr. Goldstein that you have had all you can take for one day.

WHY DOESN'T THE SAME DRUG WORK FOR EVERYONE?

Dr. Goldstein believes that FMS and CFS result from a complex interplay of genetic predisposition, developmental factors, and environmental factors. Because of the complex set of conditions accompanying onset of these diseases, Dr. Goldstein believes that the particular regions of the limbic neural network most affected and the extent and method of dysfunction to the neuronal machinery is unique enough to explain the diversity of symptoms presented and to render one drug seemingly miraculous for one patient and totally benign for another.

He also believes in the "pluripotential" of virtually all neurotransmitter substances. In other words, the patient's response depends on the cells affected, not the nature of the transmitter itself. This helps explain why the treatment response is so unique to each individual.

The success of Dr. Goldstein's treatment does not appear to correlate with either the duration or severity of your illness. Drug treatments you may have had in the past do not seem to interfere with the success of the protocol.

Dr. Goldstein equates successful treatment with "pushing the right neurochemical button." The most successful drugs Dr. Goldstein uses are *baclofen*, *nimodipine*, *gabapentin*, *oxytocin*, and intravenous *lidocaine*; the latter medication is the most effective.

IF MY TREATMENT IS SUCCESSFUL, HOW LONG WILL IT LAST?

Dr. Goldstein finds a significant problem with tolerance developing to the rapidly acting drugs in his protocol—those that exert a profound effect on regional cerebral blood flow. This tolerance can develop with as little as one dose of a medication. This "desensitization" (see Glossary) does not occur with all patients, however, any more frequently than all patients find similar benefit with a particular drug. If you do develop tolerance, Dr. Goldstein may modify the dose, try a different drug, or use inositol to reverse the developed tolerance. If memory is a problem for you, a dramatic remedy may occur in short order—with benefits lasting as long as you continue the therapy.

WHAT HAPPENS WHEN I LEAVE DR. GOLDSTEIN'S CARE?

If you have found a medication(s) that works for you, Dr. Goldstein will give you either samples or prescriptions to take with you. You may choose to return to the office if you can, or you may stay in contact with Dr. Goldstein by phone. If you are an out-of-state patient, Dr. Goldstein will work with your local primary care physician (PCP) to coordinate your continued care. This may include adjusting dosages or experimenting with new drugs in the protocol. The amount of cooperation that occurs depends largely on your PCP's openness to trying something new to help you and his or her trust in the protocol. Sharing Dr. Goldstein's book and credentials can help to establish this level of trust.

Dr. Goldstein's Theory
in a Large Nutshell

Dr. Goldstein refers to conditions as CFS, FMS, irritable bowel, and premenstrual syndrome as "neurosomatic" and believes they are disorders of central information processing with a neurologic basis. He believes that these are disorders of neural networks, resulting in functional changes in the brain, rather than physiological tissue changes. For this reason, these disorders best reveal themselves using SPECT or PET (positron emission tomography) scan imaging that reveal cerebral blood flow and metabolic functioning, respectively. Dr. Goldstein believes that actual structural deficits are uncommon in neurosomatic patients and that the disorders lie in problems with regulation of neurochemical receptors and secondary chemical messengers (those released from bound receptors). This dysregulation deprives the organism of its natural "neural plasticity," the amazing capacity of neurons and their networks to respond to changing internal and external environments.

Dr. Goldstein has advanced his theory into the pathophysiology of neurosomatic disorders to include not only dysfunction of the limbic system itself, but also dysregulation of widely distributed neural networks that regulate the limbic system, including the prefrontal cortex (PFC) basal ganglia, thalamus, and heteromodal association areas (within the PFC). Dr. Goldstein believes there are many "sensory gates" that might be dysfunctional.

Chronic fatigue syndrome manifests itself physiologically in myriad ways. It is unknown which is the fundamental starting point, if indeed there is one. Functionally, dysregulation is apparent in the dorsolateral prefrontal cortex (DLPFC)-hippocampal circuit, resulting primarily in "experiential" misinterpretations of sensory input, e.g., have I seen this before or not? In neurosomatic patients, the answer is often "no," which is often incorrect. This results in the additional stress and distraction of having to devise new behavioral strategies for stimuli incorrectly perceived as "new," rather than recognizing them as "known" stimuli for which routine behavior is appropriate.

Dysfunction of the prefrontal cortex (PFC) is also evident. Although the exact etiology of PFC dysfunction is uncertain, it is probably a combination of genetic, developmental, and environmental factors. The PFC "gates" sensory input for saliency (relevance) by comparing it to experiences and attitudes. When this gating malfunctions, unimportant stimuli make it through at the expense of input with survival value. Other input is weighted inappropriately. Inappropriate responses tend to result: light touch is painful, benign odors are noxious, and hypersentivities develop to chemicals, drugs, noise, bright lights, food, etc. The PFC also regulates the secretion of the excitatory amino acid glutamate (GT). With insufficient glutamate secretion, which occurs in neurosomatic disorders, decreased levels of other neurotransmitters, particularly norepinephrine (NE), result.

NE is paramount in the processing of sensory input due to its role in enhancing the "signal-to-noise (STN) ratio." With a high STN ratio, the organism can screen out irrelevant stimuli and accurately perceive and process input of survival value. Neurosomatic patients have a low STN ratio and often have the feeling of being bombarded with input and being unable to focus. The pathophysiology that causes this NE deficit, "noradrenergic denervation hypersensitivity," is evident in many brain sites: reduced function of the locus ceruleus (LC), which produces NE; decreased cell numbers in the LC itself that could have a similar effect on NE production; decreased secretion of glutamate from the PFC, which in turn results in low levels of NE production; or possible low levels of NE and other transmitter substances as a result of a chronic viral infection.

Substance P (SP), the "pain neurotransmitter," is another key player in neurosomatic disorders. SP has an inverse relationship with NE. When NE is low, as it is for neurosomatic patients, SP should be high, which it is–three times the normal levels in the cerebrospinal fluid of FMS patients. While NE enhances the signal-to-noise (STN) ratio, SP lowers it. High levels of SP contribute to the difficulty CFS/FMS patients have screening out irrelevant stimuli. SP also "widens receptive fields." This may account for the common progression of FMS from a regional myofascial pain problem to a diffuse, bodywide syndrome.

The role of endothelin (ET) is still uncertain, but the fact that it is the most powerful vasoconstrictor in the body, and found in excess in the cerebrospinal fluid (CSF) of FMS patients, suggests some responsibility for the symptoms associated with baseline decreases in regional cerebral blood flow (rCBF) found in CFS/FMS patients. Endothelin stimulates secretion of substance P, which is also found in excess in the CSF of FMS patients.

Dr. Goldstein also believes that neuropeptide Y (NPY) and oxytocin (OXT) deficits play a role in neurosomatic disorders.

The base neurochemical deficit, however, probably resides at the level of the prefrontal cortex, where neurons secrete excitatory amino acids (EAAs), especially glutamate, to regulate the production of biogenic amines, particularly dopamine (DA) and norepinephrine (NE). A deficiency in EAA neurotransmission, especially involving glutamate, results in impaired production of nitric oxide (NO). NO is critical to the process of long-term potentiation (LTP), or memory encoding, by increasing synaptic strength and convergence.

Because of the central deficiency of NE production, Dr. Goldstein's pharmacologic approach is to enhance the glutamate-evoked NE secretion from the locus ceruleus, possibly via the dorsal and ventral noradrenergic bundles, and the superior cervical ganglion (SCG). Figure 1 may help you to visualize the previous discussion.

DRUG THERAPIES: THE VASODILATION vs. VASOCONSTRICTION CONUNDRUM

Through many drug trials with many patients, Dr. Goldstein has uncovered a number of drugs that, for reasons still uncertain, result in a rapid, profound relief of most, if not all, of a patient's CFS/FMS symptoms. This effect occurs in 95 percent of Dr. Goldstein's patients.

Some of the medications Dr. Goldstein uses have a direct effect on centrally mediated processes (those directed by the brain). Other medications, which cross the blood-brain barrier poorly, act peripherally to indirectly affect these central processes. The latter agents can have dramatic effects on cerebral blood flow and seem to alter brain function by "stimulating peripheral nerves, autonomic ganglia, or circumventricular organs" (Goldstein, 1996, p. 155). Interestingly, acupuncture also exerts its effects on the body in this way.

FIGURE 1

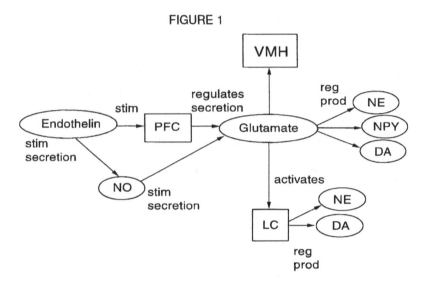

All of Dr. Goldstein's therapies attempt to modulate brain function. Oddly, some of the drugs seem to exert an effect that is the opposite of their designed intention. CFS/FMS patients have markedly reduced global and regional cerebral blood flow, known as hypoperfusion. Some of these drugs usually have a vasodilatory mode of action in the brain (opening blood vessels to increase blood flow). One would expect them to *improve* the hypoperfusion. However, when you view the brain on SPECT scan after treatment, the hypoperfusion is worse! This is true for all of the drugs in the protocol that result in rapid relief of CFS/FMS symptoms. Dr. Goldstein believes that this is because the effectiveness of the drug is not dependent on reversing the hypoperfusion at all, and that post-treatment reduction in rCBF relates less to the drug itself and more to vasoconstrictor substances released along with it. Interestingly, when a patient does not experience relief with one of these drugs, there is little to no change in their rCBF.

There exists a direct correlation between cerebral blood flow and cerebral function, so that decreased blood flow in an area of the brain equates to reduced function.

Interestingly, while one might assume that this reduction in rCBF is harmful, such may not necessarily be the case. PET studies have shown that a group of normal women experiencing transient "happiness" showed reduced rCBF while transient sadness produced the opposite–increased rCBF, albeit neither occurred in the same regions of the brain affected in CFS/FMS patients.

A NEUROCHEMICAL EXPLANATION

Dr. Goldstein proposes that the drugs that cause rapidly acting, global relief of CFS/FMS symptoms, along with epiphenomenon of reduced rCBF, exert their effects by stimulating the release of norepinephrine and possibly neuropeptide Y with which it is co-localized. After NE and NPY increase, they appear to trigger the secretion of corticotropin-releasing hormone (CRH) and inhibit the secretion of substance P. It is also possible that the stimulation of CRH secretion occurs directly.

Both NE and NPY may be responsible for the reduced rCBF evident on post-treatment SPECT scans since both are vasoconstrictors. The CRH release that follows may cause vasconstriction directly or do so indirectly by stimulating the release of NE. A contributory factor may also be that endothelial cells can synthesize and release inhibitors to nitric oxide (NO) production, the primary vasodilator in the brain, thus resulting in further vasoconstriction. Endothelin (ET) probably plays a role, as well, since it is the most powerful vasoconstrictor in the body. However, if ET stimulates SP, this fact does not explain reduced SP levels after treatment if, indeed, such is the case. Perhaps lowered SP levels are more closely linked to increased levels of NE since they are inversely proportional.

Explaining the rapid amelioration of symptoms experienced with drugs in the protocol is equally complex. The inhibition of the pain transmitter substance P has obvious benefits. Its decline probably relates to its inverse relationship with NE levels, which are higher. Increases in NE cause an increase in the signal-to-noise ratio, allowing for efficient screening of irrelevant stimuli and increasing the ability to focus and concentrate. Increased NE can improve alertness, enhance memory, and properly regulate many processes of the autonomic nervous system. Increases in NPY can improve sleep, reduce anxiety, and stimulate appetite. Increased levels of the immunosuppressive CRH can "deactivate" the immune response in CFS patients, eliminating chronic sore throats, swollen lymph nodes, low-grade fever, and other symptoms. Increased CRH also allows the hypothalamus to properly regulate core body temperature.

The mechanism of CRH increase is still uncertain. SP inhibits CRH, so with SP lowered, CRH might rise. Oxytocin (OXT) and possibly nitric oxide (NO) stimulate the release of CRH, so these neurotransmitters may play a role.

Helping You Understand
Dr. Goldstein's Book

Dr. Goldstein's book, *Betrayal By The Brain: The Neurologic Basis of Chronic Fatigue Syndrome, Fibromyalgia Syndrome, and Related Neural Network Disorders*, can be a daunting treatise to the layperson as well as a challenge for the physician who is not versed in neurology, psychiatry, immunology, and endocrinology—all specialty fields in their own right.

In reading Dr. Goldstein's book, it becomes apparent that he has drawn upon the research findings of many of his colleagues and, along with his extensive clinical experience of over 12 years and 4,000 patients, has synthesized what he refers to as an "integrative hypothesis" to suggest the pathophysiology of both fibromyalgia and chronic fatigue syndromes.

Here we will try to present enough of the salient points of the book so that you can understand the underlying concepts. We will also offer a Glossary of words and acronyms you will come across frequently as you read the book.

To the layperson, probably the most compelling evidence lies within Dr. Goldstein's case reports. It becomes less important for the suffering patient to understand why the drug protocol works, but simply that it does work for so many people.

To begin an understanding of Dr. Goldstein's theories, it is important to understand the roles of brain structures and the neurochemicals that interplay to create the complex constellation of symptoms we know as CFS and FMS.

First, we will describe the proper role and function of each brain structure or neural assembly that plays a role in neurosomatic disorders, and then we will describe its apparent dysfunction. Where applicable, we will mention drug therapies that Dr. Goldstein has found to modulate the functioning of these structures or networks to produce symptom relief. All drug names appear in italics.

Understanding the following terms will help as you read about the various structures of the brain. This nomenclature describes the location of brain structures in relation to one another.

Dorsal: pertaining to the back or posterior

Ventral: pertaining to the front or anterior

Lateral: pertaining to the side (right or left) of the median plane

Superior: situated above

Inferior: situated below

BRAIN STRUCTURES

Amygdala

Normal Function—Part of the limbic system, the amygdala is a small mass of gray matter lying in the roof of a lateral ventricle (see Glossary). The job of the amygdala is to receive input from the neocortex (the dorsal [posterior] region of the cortex) and to integrate external events with internal signals. The amygdala is also important in memory encoding, particularly for the ability to recall facts.

The amygdala's role in auditory fear conditioning is a subject of recent study. Auditory stimuli reach the acoustic thalamus and travel from there to the lateral amygdala (LA) directly or through the specialized auditory cortex within the cerebral cortex. The LA receives data through connections from the hippocampus regarding the "context" (i.e., the environmental and experiential factors surrounding the input), which helps shape the organism's response. The arbiter of this response is the dorsolateral prefrontal cortex (DLPFC). This contextualized input with DLPFC interpretation then continues from the LA to the central nucleus of the amygdala (CE) for processing. The CE then projects to the areas of the brainstem that control the response of the hippocampus, resulting in both voluntary and involuntary actions by the organism. The CE also projects to the paraventricular nucleus of the hypothalamus (PVN), another component of the limbic system. The PVN is responsible for the release of corticotropin-releasing hormone (CRH), which stimulates the release of cortisol through its regulation of adreno-corticotropic hormone (ACTH).

Dysfunction in CFS/FMS–The prefrontal cortex (PFC) regulates amygdalar input and output. A certain location within the PFC, the DLPFC, appears dysregulated. The DLPFC misinterprets the con-textualized input coming from the amygdala and hippocampus and perceives it as a novel cognitive situation rather than a known cognitive routine, resulting in an inappropriate stress response.

Decreased secretion of glutamate from the prefrontal cortex to the lateral amygdala may result in a decrease of corticotropin-releasing hormone (CRH) levels in the central nucleus of the amygdala.

When negative outcomes become expected and the subsequent arousal from fear and threat becomes chronic, depression and/or anxiety usually follow, accompanied by activation of the hypotha-lamic-pituitary-adrenal (HPA) axis and elevation of stress hormones such as cortisol. This expectation of fearful events causes activation

Brain structures appear in boxes; neurochemicals in ellipses.

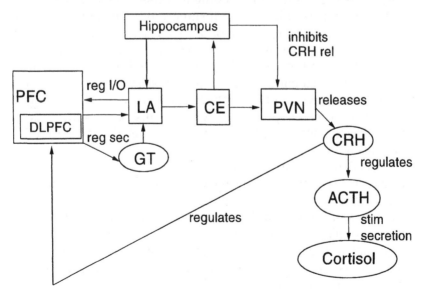

of the amygdala. In disorders such as depression, schizophrenia, and obsessive-compulsive disorder (OCD), *increased* CRH levels in the central nucleus of the amygdala accompany this activation, setting the stage for chronic arousal and its deleterious effects. The amygdala, brainstem, and hypothalamus comprise the neural network that activates the CE CRH release, facilitated by substances called glucocorticoids (such as cortisol). Chronically elevated levels of glucocorticoids (like cortisol) can damage hippocampal neurons, producing further levels of PVN CRH because they alter the ability of the hippocampus to inhibit levels of CRH. Obviously, another mechanism must be at work in neurosomatic disorders in which CRH levels are *low*. (See the section on the hippocampus for Dr. Goldstein's theory.)

Basal Ganglia

Normal Function–These groups of nerve cells sit above the brainstem and next to the limbic system in each hemisphere of the brain. The caudate nucleus, which is part of the basal ganglia, together with the cerebellum, helps maintain balance and coordinate complex body movements, including starting and stopping motion and producing smooth, flowing muscular action. The basal ganglia also play a role in encoding procedural, or skill memory.

Along with its role in coordinating motor functions, the basal ganglia may be the most important structure for nociception (the mechanism by which we perceive painful stimuli). The basal ganglia processes information about noxious and nonnoxious sensory stimuli. The basal ganglia receive this information from nociceptive neurons that cover wide receptive fields, sometimes including the entire body (unlike specialized sense organs such as the eyes and ears). These neurons carry information about the intensity of the stimulus but not its location.

Specialized neurons within the striatum of the basal ganglia may act as sensory gates and contribute to the determination of information saliency and the corresponding motor response.

Studies of injuries to the structures of the basal ganglia demonstrate its link to mood regulation. In most of these disorders, like Parkinson's disease, a motor disorder often accompanied by pain and depression, lack of dopamine plays a major role, along with low levels of serotonin and norepinephrine.

The caudate nucleus of the basal ganglia and the orbitofrontal cortex (OFC) are the primary anatomical structures involved in producing slow-wave-sleep.

*Dysfunction in CFS/FMS—*Hypoperfusion (reduced cerebral blood flow) is evident in the right caudate nucleus of neurosomatic patients. There is a direct correlation between the degree of hypoperfusion and the patient's level of pain.

Because of the wide receptive fields of neurons within the basal ganglia, it is possible that they play a role in the diffuse, bodywide pain perception of FMS.

A very complex neural network loop appears to exist, with relevance to cognitive function, connecting the prefrontal cortex (PFC), the structures of the basal ganglia, and the thalamus. It is the CSTC, or cortico-striatalthalamo-cortical loop. Stated very simplistically, in neurosomatic disorders, reduced function of the PFC and caudate nucleus of the basal ganglia combine with increased inhibition in the thalamus to decrease "thalamocortical excitation." Dysregulation of glutamate, gamma-amino butyric acid (GABA), and dopamine all play a part. Dr. Goldstein speculates that this reduced "thalamocortical excitation" may be the underlying cause of neurosomatic disorders.

Problems with mood regulation are a major component of neurosomatic disorders and the basal ganglia may be the locus of control. Both depression and mania have a link to reduced function of the caudate nucleus. Injury to the structures of the basal ganglia can cause apathy, depression, mania, uninhibited behavior, obsessive-compulsive-disorder, Tourette's syndrome, irritability, and amnesia, among other symptoms. Interestingly, however, many CFS/FMS patients do not experience depression, and disorders falling within the obsessive-compulsive spectrum are uncommon. From a functional standpoint, in many respects, OCD's are the opposite of CFS/FMS.

Reduced dopamine levels in the cerebrospinal fluid are likely due to reduced glutamate secretion from the PFC to the ventral tegmental area (VTA) of the caudate nucleus that releases dopamine. Reduced dopamine levels in the VTA may produce anxiety.

A dysfunction in the caudate nucleus of the basal ganglia could affect the onset and duration of restorative slow-wave sleep, a common problem in neurosomatic disorders.

Drug Remediation–The use of dopamine agonists (drugs designed to increase levels of dopamine or prevent its reuptake) are ineffective in neurosomatic patients.

Cerebellum

Normal Function–Located just below and outside the cerebral hemispheres and behind the brainstem, the cerebellum, or "small brain," is the center for the control and coordination of movement. The cerebellum monitors a "map" of the body's position and location and controls the process of "proprioception," by which the body knows where it is and where it is going. Through its connections to the brainstem, the cerebellum receives information from receptors in the skin, muscles, joints, tendons, and the balance mechanisms of the inner ears. When the central nervous system orders a movement to occur, the cerebral cortex activates a "program" of learned patterns of motion carried within the cerebellum. The cerebellum then continuously monitors the body, particularly its posture and state of muscle contraction or relaxation. Working with the caudate nucleus that is part of the basal ganglia, the cerebellum then corrects any discrepancies between the "program" and what the body is actually doing, producing smoothly coordinated body movements and maintaining posture and balance. The cerebellum also plays a role in encoding procedural, or skill, memory.

The above description represents the traditional, textbook view of the cerebellum as a motor mechanism. However, when viewed with functional brain imaging, the cerebellum is also active during cognitive and language tasks. The neodentate, a recently evolved part of the cerebellum, which has grown very large in humans, has as its target structures the brainstem, thalamus, and the cerebral cortex. Its primary target, however, is the frontal lobe, particularly the dorsolateral prefrontal cortex (DLPFC) and Broca's language area in the inferior prefrontal cortex. Broca's area is active in the process of word finding, a function often difficult for CFS/FMS patients. Two-way communications exist between the cortex and the cerebellum, facilitating coordination in performing cognitive and language tasks. Studies imply that the neodentate performs "counting, timing, sequencing, predicting and anticipatory planning, error detecting and correction, shifting of attention, pattern generation, adaption, and learning" (Goldstein, 1996, p. 97); many of the functions impaired in neurosomatic disorders.

Dysfunction in CFS/FMS–PET scan (functional brain imaging) has revealed baseline hypometabolism (reduced metabolism) in certain locations within the cerebellum.

Generally, Dr. Goldstein has not seen evidence of cerebellar dysfunction, either through functional PET scanning or SPECT scanning in CFS/FMS patients; however, he believes that the cerebellum and its associated neural network are likely contributors to the cognitive difficulties found in neurosomatic disorders.

Dr. Goldstein conceives of hypofunction (reduced function) occurring in the cerebellar-locus ceruleus pathway of CFS/FMS patients, due to reduced LC function, resulting in difficulty filtering out irrelevant sensory stimuli.

Cerebral Cortex

Normal Function–The outer layer of the brain, the deeply convoluted cerebral cortex known as "gray matter," makes up about 40 percent of the brain's total weight. One of the functions of this region is to store memories. The cortex is divided into two hemispheres connected by the corpus callosum, allowing an individual to function as a coordinated whole. There are specific regions of the cortex associated with certain senses: the sensory cortex receives signals from the skin, bones, joints, and muscles, producing the sensations of touch and pressure; the visual cortex receives signals from the optic nerve; other less specific cortical regions receive signals regarding hearing, smell, and taste sensations.

In addition to sensory areas, there is also a motor cortex that activates the muscles. Not all movements initiate from the cortex, however. Some well-learned patterns of motion, such as that required for walking, are the responsibility of the cerebellum. When the central nervous system gives the command to "walk," the cerebral cortex activates the walking "program," and the cerebellum takes over. It compares what the muscles and joints are actually doing to the program instructions, and with help from the caudate nucleus, it corrects any discrepancies. This frees the cortex to deal with newly acquired, skilled movements.

Linked to the clearly defined sensory and motor areas are "association areas." These association areas, comprising almost three-quarters of the cerebral cortex in both hemispheres, perform comprehension and recognition functions, put factual memories into context for efficient storage and retrieval, do arithmetic, and are the seats of thinking, decision making, and emotional experience.

The two hemispheres of the cerebral cortex specialize in processing very different information. The left hemisphere usually dominates, controlling our speech and language, the ability to read and write, and the use of our dominant hand. It is also the site of our analytical, sequential task-oriented, and symbolic activities, including math, logic, and reasoning. The right hemisphere processes visual, spatial, and emotional information and is responsible for our artistic inclinations and for recognizing faces. The left hemisphere seems to operate with working memory and behavior already in context, i.e., our normal routines. The right hemisphere, by contrast, deals with new situations presented from the external environment and develops new, context-independent behaviors. From a biochemical standpoint, dopamine (DA) pathways predominate to the left hemisphere, and norepinephrine (NE) pathways predominate to the right. NE is essential to cognitive novelty and DA to cognitive routines.

Dysfunction in CFS/FMS–An explanation for the diffuse, body-wide pain of FMS may be a malfunction in the right hemisphere of the brain. The right hemisphere processes output from neurons with large, overlapping receptive fields, whereas the left hemisphere processes output from small receptive-field neurons.

Performing math functions should activate the left parietal lobe of the brain. However, when a CFS patient performs math, a SPECT scan shows activation of the right hemisphere, particularly the right DLPFC. The DLPFC should handle novel stimuli, and math is clearly in the domain of the left brain as a routine cognitive function. This demonstrates one of the main dysfunctions of CFS: a misperception of cognitive novelty. This could result in perceiving previously benign events as new and stressful and explain the anxiety that is often concomitant with CFS.

CFS patients also appear to have abnormal sensory processing of sound, believed to occur in the DLPFC-hippocampal-auditory cortex circuit.

Dorsolateral Prefrontal Cortex (DLPFC)

Normal Function–An area of the PFC, located dorsally (toward the back) and laterally (to the sides), the dorsolateral prefrontal cortex (DLPFC) performs "executive functions," and may be the most important heteromodal association area for new learning. The DLPFC "controls organization, planning activities that involve sequential tasks, motivation and drive, self-analysis, and neural regulation. The DLPFC is also involved in memory encoding, or the making of new memories" (Goldstein, 1996, p. 50).

Dysfunction in CFS/FMS–Hypofunction (reduced function) of the DLPFC is consistent across the CFS patient population. Hypoperfusion (reduced rCBF) of the DFPLC occurs most frequently in the right hemisphere of CFS/FMS patients.

The DLPFC may be the most important heteromodal association area of all in the context of neurosomatic disorders. Its job is to watch and evaluate the activities of cognitive networks and to choose a proper response, using input from the limbic system. If processing of this sensory input is incorrect in the first place, then the decision made by the DLPFC may be inappropriate. This can explain symptoms such as pain and weakness with no physiologic basis and problems with temperature control and weight maintenance (independent of diet).

Right DLPFC dysfunction in neurosomatic disorders may result in input from the amygdala and hippocampus being incorrectly interpreted as previously unseen and undealt with (i.e., not a part of our known cognitive routines–the domain of the left hemisphere). This misinterpretation can produce anxiety and an inappropriate stress response.

The PFC may be responsible for maintaining chronic central pain syndromes. If an individual experiences an injury that resolves itself over time, the DLPFC may integrate these physical and mental "images" permanently, i.e., the microneural assembly may not remodel itself to reflect the new state of the organism. Given its function in synthesizing new behaviors from previous "context," the DLPFC could also be responsible for the placebo effect, yet another disorder of information processing.

Memory encoding and problem solving occur in the DLPFC-hippo-campal circuit. Impairments of both functions exist in CFS. The DLPFC may be responsible for gating the hippocampus by virtue of altering secretion of glutamate (input) or changing NO production (output). Glutamate levels may be deficient in the DLPFC of CFS patients.

Hippocampus

Normal Function—Part of the limbic system, the process of long-term potentiation (LTP), or memory encoding, occurs here. Nitric oxide (NO) secreted by endothelial cells acts as a "retrograde neu-rotransmitter" to enhance the presynaptic activity of neurons in-volved in LTP in the hippocampus and the neocortex. NO is se-creted from the post-synaptic neuron then diffuses back, in a retrograde fashion, into the firing, presynaptic neuron that is al-ready releasing its neurotransmitter. At the presynaptic neuron, NO stimulates glutamate secretion that "potentiates" the synaptic con-nection, allowing a stronger signal to pass. NO may also increase "synaptic convergence," a process by which an individual neuron has stronger connections with fewer target cells. See diagram (page 54) under GLUTAMATE in the Neurotransmitter section for further information and clarification.

Some types of short–term memories made in the hippocampus strengthen during slow-wave sleep (SWS) by repeated neuronal firings in the hippocampus. REM sleep also plays a role in consoli-dating new memories.

Dysfunction in CFS/FMS—Hypofunction of the hippocampus is common in CFS patients.

Excess secretion of cortisol (a glucocorticoid) may damage hip-pocampal neurons during times of prolonged stress. Altered regula-tion of corticosteroid receptors in the hippocampus that handle the excess cortisol may also occur. Excess secretion of cortisol during stress could cause the glucocorticoid receptors in the hippocampus to become upregulated (i.e., increased in numbers), binding more and more cortisol. With this cortisol bound to receptors in the hip-pocampus, the hippocampus might further inhibit the paraventricu-lar nucleus of the hypothalamus (PVN) from producing any more

CRH since CRH regulates the secretion of cortisol. This could account for the low levels of CRH found in CFS/FMS patients.

Reduced and disrupted sleep cycles (especially SWS) in CFS provide an explanation for the difficulty these patients have in making new memories. Insufficient glutamate secretion from the presynaptic neuron impairs the synaptic strengthening required for long-term potentiation.

Memory encoding and problem solving occur in the DLPFC-hippocampal circuit. Impairments of both functions exist in CFS. The DLPFC may be responsible for gating the hippocampus by virtue of altering secretion of glutamate (input) or changing NO production (output).

Drug Remediation–Nimodipine, a central nervous system (CNS) calcium channel blocker, may restore the proper regulation of corticosteroid receptors in the hippocampus. *Nimodipine* may also increase the neuronal plasticity of the hippocampal network by increasing the neuronal firing rate.

Hypothalamic-Pituitary Axis (HPA AXIS)

*Normal Function–*The HPA axis is a neural network consisting of the hypothalamus and the pituitary and adrenal glands.

*Dysfunction in CFS/FMS–*Much work exists on the effect of stressors occurring during the neonatal and early development stages of an organism to the HPA axis. HPA dysfunction may result in an increase in somatic symptoms into adulthood, decreased CRH production, reduced and abnormal CRH receptors in the limbic system, and increased responsiveness of the HPA axis to stress. Dr. Goldstein believes that these stressors occurring early in development (or later with the addition of a triggering factor) can interact with genetic predisposition factors to cause altered prefrontal cortex (PFC) function resulting in misjudgments of information salience that control this sensory gating. He sees this function mediated by circuits between the hippocampus and the paraventricular nucleus of the hypothalamus (PVN). The PVN controls the production of corticotropin-releasing hormone (CRH), which controls the secretion of cortisol by its regulation of adrenocorticotropic hormone (ACTH). Cortisol levels increase with stress. CRH levels, which are low in CFS/FMS patients, influence the proper functioning of three major gating areas: the PFC itself, the locus ceruleus (LC), and the superior cervical ganglion (SCG).

Interestingly, primate studies have shown that subjects who are unable to differentiate harmless situations from threatening ones have the highest levels of cortisol, whereas those with an outlet for their aggression, those with a variety of beneficial relationships, and those who interpret correctly the outcome of win/lose situations have the lowest cortisol levels.

Dr. Goldstein believes that behavioral and neuroimmunoendocrine disorders in adulthood could be the result of an inappropriate reaction to stress (either a depressed response or hypervigilance on the part of the HPA axis), particularly if accompanied by a dysfunction in the PFC that results in an evaluation of nonstressful stimuli as stressful. Deleterious chronic HPA axis activation may occur when a patient perceives lack of control over symptoms, lack of predictability of those symptoms, does not have enough protective relationships, and does not have a sense that things are getting better rather than worse.

Hypothalamus

Normal Function–Part of the limbic system, in an area of the forebrain above the brainstem, the hypothalamus is located under the thalamus and above the pituitary gland. The hypothalamus is the command center, coordinating the activities of our nervous and endocrine (hormonal) systems. The hypothalamus controls our sympathetic nervous system–part of the autonomic nervous system (see Glossary). The sympathetic nervous system activates under stress or excitement and produces what we know as the "fight-or-flight response." It causes increased heartbeat and breathing, widens the pupils, increases blood flow to the muscles, and restricts blood flow to the skin and digestive system. Also concerned with maintaining internal body temperature, the hypothalamus may cause us to sweat or shiver in response to changing temperatures. The hypothalamus also stimulates our appetite for food and drink when it receives signals that our glucose levels in the blood and our body's water content are too low. Controlling our circadian rhythms, the hypothalamus also controls cycles of body temperature, blood pressure, hormone levels, and much more. The hypothalamus also regulates sleep, sexual arousal, and our mood and emotions.

The hypothalamus controls the release of hormones from the pituitary gland. It does this directly, through a short stalk of nerve fibers connected to the pituitary, and indirectly, through the secretion of hormones called "releasing factors," which flow to the pituitary. Through this indirect method, the hypothalamus can control endocrine organs other than the pituitary, including the thyroid, adrenal cortex, and gonads.

It may also be the hypothalamus that provides part of the biological link between the nervous and immune systems. Damage to the hypothalamus can affect the activity of lymphocytes, the body's white cell defense system.

Dysfunction in CFS/FMS–For additional information, reference the section on the paraventricular nucleus of the hypothalamus (PVN), which is responsible for the release of the corticotropin-releasing hormone (CRH). CRH levels are low in CFS/FMS patients. CRH levels influence the proper functioning of three major sensory gating areas: the prefrontal cortex (PFC), the locus ceruleus (LC) and the superior cervical ganglion (SCG). This emphasizes its role in neurosomatic disorders.

Drug Remediation–Known best as a local anesthetic, *lidocaine*, when given intravenously, will act in the hypothalamus to increase secretion of central CRH.

Limbic System

Normal Function–Lying beneath the cerebral cortex and forming the inner border of the two cerebral hemispheres are the nerve centers of the limbic system. They include the hypothalamus, hippocampus, amygdala, fornix, and olfactory bulb. Together, they play a role in the autonomic nervous system, controlling automatic body functions such as the basic drives for food, sex, and survival, as well as maintenance of the body's internal environment. The limbic system is also integral to emotion, the sense of smell, and the consolidation of memories, particularly factual memories. Smells can evoke such nostalgia because the olfactory receptors are actual neurons connecting directly to the limbic system–the seat of emotion, memory, and sexuality.

The limbic neural network is like a computer, receiving input from the inside and outside environments, processing that input by integrating it with experiences and attitudes, then producing an output response, which should maximize the individual's potential for survival. "The limbic system is a high order functional regulator (integrative processing) in the brain, and has effects on fatigue, pain, sleep, weight, appetite, libido, respiration, temperature, blood pressure, memory, attention, concept formation, mood, vigilance, the immune and endocrine systems, and the modulation of the peripheral nervous system (to name a few)" (Goldstein, 1996, p. 20).

Dysfunction in CFS/FMS–Dysfunction of the limbic system may take the form of a maladaptive response to stress or aberrant processing of sensory input. "Sensory gating" is the weight, or importance, given to any sensory input. Inappropriate weighting of stimuli may lead to sound, light, and smell hypersensitivity in CFS/FMS patients.

Pain, a major factor in FMS, CFS, IBS (irritable bowel syndrome), and migraine headache, is probably under central control and therefore subject to dysregulation in a malfunctioning neural network. There are numerous descending inhibitory pathways for pain that lead from the brainstem as well as from higher centers, including the limbic system, the thalamus, and the cerebral cortex. The muscle fatigue of CFS (and likely FMS) is also under central regulation.

During exercise stress studies, CFS/FMS patients had an irregularity in tidal volume (the amount of air inspired and expired). In normal controls, the tidal volume increases linearly and then levels off when it reaches maximal tidal volume. In the patient group, particularly those with both CFS and FMS, the tidal volume was erratic. This points clearly to limbic system dysfunction since automatic respiration is under its control.

Brain SPECT scans have demonstrated abnormal regional cerebral blood flow (rCBF) in both CFS and FMS patients. Both have regional hypoperfusion (reduced blood flow), more pronounced in the right hemisphere than in the left, with FMS patients having more severe hypoperfusion. In exercise stress studies, one would expect rCBF to increase; in CFS/FMS patients, it decreases. This is another function under the control of the limbic system.

Panic disorder may operate under a primarily limbic system mechanism. In family studies in which parents or siblings also have CFS/FMS, the occurrence of panic disorder correlates most highly.

The limbic system is the primary mediator of the stress response. It is possible that long-lasting functional changes may be occurring in the neurons of this network, perhaps damaged by excessive cortisol secretion during prolonged stress. The damage may be more far-reaching than just the transmitters and receptors and may include many secondary chemical messengers, including hormones. Probably some stressor initially triggers CFS/FMS in predisposed individuals: child abuse, viral infections, surgery, extreme overexertion (physical or mental), childbirth, or a highly emotional event.

Locus Ceruleus (LC)

Normal Function–Part of the brainstem, the locus ceruleus is the manufacturing site for much of the norepinephrine (NE) in the brain.

Dysfunction in CFS/FMS–The locus ceruleus probably hypofunctions in CFS, possibly resulting in an impairment of the process by which the signal-to-noise (STN) ratio increases. When the STN process is functioning effectively, screening of sensory input allows only stimuli of value to go through to the organism. The NE-releasing fibers of the LC suppress weak inputs and intensify strong inputs, enhancing the ability to separate relevant and irrelevant stimuli. A dysfunction in this filtering process could result in ADD (attention deficit disorder) and the common complaint CFS patients have about freeways and shopping malls–a feeling that too much is going on at once.

Studies reveal that stress-resistant organisms have higher levels of activity in the locus ceruleus than stress-susceptible individuals. This is consistent with the reduced function shown in the LC of CFS patients. Stress susceptibility may be the result of decreased CRH and decreased PFC glutamate input to the locus ceruleus, which would result in lower levels of norepinephrine. Stress-susceptible individuals also show a lower number of LC cell numbers, perhaps related to the reduced LC function in CFS patients.

LC dysfunction can also cause decreases in dopamine levels in the PFC.

Excitatory amino acids (EAAs) activate the LC. Reduced LC function may be explainable by reduced EAA (particularly glutamate) secretion from the prefrontal cortex (PFC). Deficiencies in EAA neurotransmission could also result in impaired production of nitric oxide (NO). NO is a retrograde neurotransmitter that functions with glutamate to strengthen synaptic connections during the critical process of encoding new memories.

Drug Remediation–The LC, due to its production of the vasoconstrictor norepinephrine (NE), likely contributes to the marked reduction in rCBF seen in Dr. Goldstein's rapidly acting CFS/FMS treatments.

Drugs that would increase the production of norepinephrine in the locus ceruleus could have the effect of decreasing anxiety and most other neurosomatic symptoms.

Because of the central deficiency of NE production, Dr. Goldstein's pharmacologic approach is to enhance the glutamate-evoked NE secretion from the locus ceruleus, possibly via the dorsal and ventral noradrenergic bundles, and the superior cervical ganglion (SCG).

Nefazodone, *pindolol*, and *risperidone* all act to increase the glutamate-evoked secretion of NE from the locus ceruleus.

Orbitofrontal Cortex (OFC)

Normal Function–Part of the prefrontal cortex, the orbitofrontal cortex (OFC), allows selective sifting of environmental stimuli, allowing through only those stimuli of relevance to the organism.

The OFC also modulates the secretion of dopamine in the striatum of the basal ganglia. Dopamine is a critical neurotransmitter in establishing cognitive routines.

The OFC, along with the caudate nucleus of the basal ganglia, are the primary anatomical structures involved in producing slow-wave sleep (SWS).

Dysfunction in CFS/FMS–A dysfunction in the OFC could affect the onset and duration of restorative, slow-wave sleep, a common problem in neurosomatic disorders.

Paraventricular Nucleus of the Hypothalamus (PVN)

Normal Function–The PVN of the hypothalamus, another component of the limbic system, has projections from the central nucleus of the amygdala (CE). The PVN is responsible for the release of corti-cotropin-releasing hormone (CRH), which in turn stimulates the release of cortisol through its regulation of the adrenocorticotropic hormone (ACTH). Cortisol secretion increases with stress.

Dysfunction in CFS/FMS–Certain stress conditions can result in diminished release of CRH from the PVN. CRH levels are low in neurosomatic patients.

Prefrontal Cortex (PFC)

Normal Function–Part of the cerebral cortex and located in an area of the frontal lobes just behind the forehead, the PFC makes "associations" and seems to be the basis for our intellectual achievements. The PFC comes into play whenever we create something that was not there before, e.g., composing music, reaching a judgment, having a new idea, planning a course of action, or even worrying about the future. The prefrontal cortex has close connections to the thalamus, the caudate nucleus in the basal ganglia, and the brainstem. This linkage to lower brain structures allows us to associate our memories with emotions and to have our memories evoke actual physical responses.

All input processed by the limbic system refers to the PFC.

The PFC is unique among regions of the brain in that it regulates its own neurotransmitter input. It projects excitatory neurons that secrete the excitatory amino acid glutamate to brainstem nuclei, causing the production of "biogenic amines," particularly dopamine (DA) and norepinephrine (NE).

In the primate brain, the PFC is the most important region for inhibiting the processing of irrelevant stimuli.

The PFC determines information "salience" after being presented with preprocessed sensory input from the internal and external environments. The jobs of the PFC are to "gate" or control what input continues beyond it to processing areas such as the hippocampus and amygdala, and to sample, or "quality check," the output from those processing centers. After receiving sensory input, the amygdala receives "contextual conditioning" information from the hippocampus, which adds a layer of environmental or experiential factors. The DLPFC provides the ultimate interpretation.

Dysfunction in CFS/FMS–Any dysfunction in the PFC can, in turn, cause problems with limbic system regulation.

The PFC modulates input and output coming from the amygdala and this process appears to be dysregulated in CFS/FMS.

Right DLPFC dysfunction in neurosomatic disorders may result in input from the amygdala and hippocampus being incorrectly interpreted as previously unseen and undealt with (i.e., not a part of our known cognitive routines–the domain of the left hemisphere). This misinterpretation can produce anxiety and an inappropriate stress response.

Dr. Goldstein postulates a glutamate deficiency as the chemical "starting point" for CFS. If the PFC secretes insufficient glutamate because of misperception of the saliency of sensory input, the result will be decreased levels of norepinephrine (and NPY with which it is co-localized) and dopamine.

Decreased secretion of PFC glutamate to the lateral amygdala (LA) may decrease CRH levels in the central nucleus of the amygdala (CE).

Neurosomatic disorders and other disorders with circadian rhythm components may relate to reduced glutamate secretion from the PFC. Secretion of NPY is also critical to maintaining circadian rhythms. Low levels of glutamate and NPY, as well as serotonin and vasoactive intestinal peptide (VIP), which potentiate the action of glutamate in this role, all contribute to circadian dysregulation.

The PFC and limbic system regulate automatic respiration. This process is often dysregulated in CFS/FMS, as shown by exercise stress studies that demonstrate highly variable tidal volume (the amount of air inspired and expired).

Drug Remediation–*Glycine* enhances glutamate transmission and may enhance its release from the PFC.

All antidepressants may provide relief for CFS/FMS sufferers by increasing extracellular dopamine in the prefrontal cortex.

Superior Cervical Ganglion (SCG)

Normal Function–The superior cervical ganglion (SCG) is one of the groups of ganglia (masses of nerve tissue apart from the brain or spinal cord) comprising the autonomic nervous system–controlling our involuntary body functions.

The SCG is an important gating area due to its secretion of NE, a neurotransmitter that increases the signal-to-noise (STN) ratio, allowing the filtering out of irrelevant stimuli.

The SCG secretes both norepinephrine (NE) and neuropeptide Y (NPY); substance P can disrupt this process. Release of endothelin, NPY and NO occurs with activation of SCG fibers associated with the sympathetic nervous system (SNS), the part of the ANS that prepares us for action.

Dysfunction in CFS/FMS–Deficiencies of glutamate and CRH may impair the functioning of the SCG. Reduced secretion of NE from the SCG impairs its sensory gating capabilities and may contribute to the central NE deficiency of neurosomatic disorders.

Drug Remediation–Because of the central deficiency of NE production, Dr. Goldstein's pharmacologic approach is to enhance NE secretion from the locus ceruleus, possibly via the dorsal and ventral noradrenergic bundles, and the superior cervical ganglion (SCG).

The SCG is a possible site of vasoconstrictor neurons that are responsible for the marked reduction in rCBF in Dr. Goldstein's rapidly acting CFS treatments. Stimulation of preganglionic cholinergic neurons (those that release acetylcholine) acting on upregulated (i.e., increased numbers of) receptors in the SCG might produce the release of NE, NPY, and ET, all of which can cause vasoconstriction, accounting for the reduced rCBF.

Pyridostigmine, while not crossing the blood-brain barrier, still increases secretion of growth hormone (GH), perhaps by its stimulation of the superior cervical ganglion (SCG).

Thalamic Reticular Nucleus (RT)

Normal Function–The thalamic reticular nucleus is a thin layer of cells wrapped around the dorsal thalamus. Providing the earliest developmental linkage between the thalamus and the cortex, the RT connects the numerous "relay nuclei" of the thalamus. The relay nuclei are the structures by which the thalamus receives sensory information from the body. The RT then regulates the transmission of pain and other signals to the cortex. The RT controls interneurons that release GABA, an inhibitory neurotransmitter whose selective secretion can send a sensory message of either pain or touch to the cortex. When the sensation is pain, GABA inhibits messages regarding touch.

The RT also provides a pathway for crosstalk between the thalamus in each hemisphere, widening its sphere of influence to include the cerebral cortex and basal ganglia on both sides of the brain. The RT may help us focus our attention as well as regulate the connections that develop between the thalamus and the cortex.

The RT plays a role in the transition from waking to sleeping by regulating the action of thalamic interneurons that release the inhibitory neurotransmitter GABA. GABA deactivates the neurons that produce excitatory neurotransmitters such as acetylcholine and glutamate, inhibiting thalamocortical neurotransmissions and allowing uninterrupted sleep and REM sleep to occur.

Dysfunction in CFS/FMS–Dysfunction in the RT, particularly related to secretion of GABA, could impede the onset of sleep as well as sleep maintenance, resulting in frequent awakenings or even nightmares.

With GABA secretion from the RT impaired, both touch and actual pain could produce the perception of pain. This could help explain the central pain mechanism of CFS/FMS.

The developmental plasticity of the RT makes it a probable structure for dysregulation in neurosomatic disorders. Inappropriate interconnections between the thalamus and the cortex might result from genetic factors or developmental and/or environmental stressors. A dysfunctional prefrontal cortex (PFC) could cause dysregulation in the RT's sensory gating functions. This could result in many of the bodily symptoms experienced by neurosomatic patients such as general pain, nerve pain, hot/cold sensations, and sleep disorders. It could also help explain the intermittent nature of these sensations and their tendency to move around the body without explanation.

The fatigue that CFS patients experience, along with their inability to focus attention, may relate to dysfunction in thalamic nuclei, because of dysregulation by the reticular nuclei and its cortical connections.

Drug Remediation–*Gabapentin* may enhance the function of the RT. *Gabapentin* increases GABA, inhibiting an inhibitory system in the RT, resulting in thalamocortical excitation.

Thalamus

Normal Function–Located above the brainstem and connected to all parts of the brain, the thalamus acts as the major relay station and processing center for messages between lower brain regions and the cerebral cortex above it–especially for information about sensations (particularly pain, temperature, and touch) and movement. The thalamus acts as a sensory filter, screening out nonessential signals and allowing concentration to be given to a task. A part of the thalamus is also important in memory encoding, particularly the ability to recall facts.

All sensory input (except smell) travels through the thalamus and then on to individual sensory cortices. From there, the association areas of the PFC as well as the hippocampus and amygdala of the limbic system provide interpretation.

Dysfunction in CFS/FMS–Hypoperfusion (reduced rCBF) is evident in both hemispheres of the thalamus.

Dr. Goldstein believes the thalamus to be the most sophisticated gating structure of the central nervous system and a potential site for sensory input abnormalities, which he believes are the cause of neurosomatic disorders.

Trigeminal Nerve

Normal Function–The fifth cranial nerve, the trigeminal nerve, arises from the area of the brainstem called the pons and splits into three branches, which in turn form a complex network of nerves. The ophthalmic nerve supplies most of the scalp, the upper eyelid, the cornea, and controls the production of tears; the maxillary nerve supplies the upper jaw; and the mandibular nerve supplies the tongue (also controlling production of saliva from the salivary glands), lower jaw, and jaw muscles that contract for chewing.

Because of the importance of the limbic system in neurosomatic disorders, Dr. Goldstein has searched for access routes and then drugs that will target the limbic system. The trigeminal nerve provides one of these pathways.

Dr. Goldstein has proposed the following routing from the trigeminal nerve to the limbic system: "I have proposed that there is a multisynaptic pathway from the mesencephalic trigeminal tract to the pontine reticular formation, and/or to the hypothalamus and thalamic reticular nuclei, and subsequently to the cortex and the limbic system, perhaps the hippocampus" (Goldstein, 1993, p. 242).

Dysfunction in CFS/FMS–There is no dysfunction in the trigeminal nerve in CFS/FMS. It provides a neural pathway for drugs to affect the brain.

Drug Remediation–Dr. Goldstein uses *naphazoline HCl*, an ophthalmic solution, one drop in each eye, to modulate the trigeminal nerve. As in all agents that cause rapid relief from CFS/FMS symptoms, *naphazoline HCl* causes reduced rCBF. Dr. Goldstein may also employ a nasal spray and *nitroglycerine* under the tongue. All of these agents have a direct pathway to the brain through the eyes, nose, and mouth.

Sumatriptan may block trigeminal nerve transmission of substance P, the pain neurotransmitter.

Ventromedial Nucleus of the Hypothalamus (VMH)

Normal Function–Part of the limbic system, the VMH is the major hypothalamic component of the sympathetic nervous system (the involuntary part that prepares us for action) and the primary controller of central energy metabolism. The VMH has a major role in regulating glucose uptake in the skeletal muscles, the heart, and in brown adipose tissue (BAT). The VMH also regulates the stress hormones, particularly glucocorticoids, including cortisol. The VMH can integrate exercise and energy metabolism simultaneously, mobilizing for exercise with release of glutamate and slowing metabolism by presynaptically inhibiting glutamate via the $GABA_A$ system.

PFC neurons may regulate the integration of exercise and energy metabolism by acting at the VMH glutamate receptors in conjunction with norepinephrine (NE).

Dysfunction in CFS/FMS–Dysfunction of the PFC-VMH neural network may be responsible for metabolic abnormalities associated with CFS, including low anaerobic threshold (the point when muscles start making energy from glucose in the absence of oxygen) and changes in the function and possibly structure of mitochondria.

VMH dysfunction may also be responsible for low levels of natural killer (NK) cells in CFS patients as well as low levels of growth hormone (GH).

Findings of unexpectedly decreased hormone levels as well as sometimes unchanged or even lower core body temperatures after exercise point to the possibility of neurohormonally mediated VMH dysfunction, probably related to corticotropin-releasing hormone (CRH). CRH is responsible for elevating core body temperature after exercise, rather than the heat generated by the exercise itself, as might be expected. The hypothalamus controls this temperature elevation, involving a change in the thermoregulatory set-point. The temperature intolerance of CFS/FMS patients may be the result of a similar mechanism gone awry.

TRANSMITTER SUBSTANCES

First, some basic definitions:

Neuron: A nerve cell. A neuron consists of a cell body and one or more branches called dendrites through which the neuron can receive impulses from other cells. Every neuron has at least one axon, a long, white-sheathed tail, which can range in length from one inch to several feet, through which the neuron can *transmit* nerve impulses. The axon forms branches at its end called terminals (as many as 10,000), which relay signals to target cells, including the dendrites of other neurons, muscle cells, or glands.

> When an impulse reaches an axon terminal, it releases a packet of message-bearing chemicals, or neurotransmitters, which jump the tiny synaptic gap and fit into protein receptors on the dendrites of the receiving cells. These neurotransmitters may serve as either excitatory or inhibitory signals: They either impel the neuron to produce an electrical impulse or prevent it from firing. Certain neurotransmitters can also modulate the sensitivity of neurons to the signals of other neurotransmitters. Each neuron keeps a running account of all the signals it receives, both excitatory and inhibitory. While in a resting state, the inside of a neuron maintains a net negative charge in

relation to the fluid that surrounds it. This salty fluid—which may be a carryover from the primordial oceans in which life began—contains a high level of positively charged sodium ions. Incoming excitatory signals change the properties of the neuron's membrane, opening tiny channels that allow the sodium ions to rush into the neuron from the extracellular fluid. This influx of positively charged ions brings the neuron closer to initiating an impulse. Inhibitory signals have the reverse effect, suppressing the neuron's tendency to fire. If the signals received by the neuron add up to sufficient excitation and the neuron reaches a sufficient excitatory threshold, it fires. The impulse then flashes down the axon, releasing packets of a specific neurotransmitter at its tip. These chemicals zip across the synaptic gap to another cell and start the process again. (Poole, 1986, pp. 339-340)

Nerve cells fall into three classifications: interneurons (forming all the interconnecting electrical circuitry within the central nervous system), motoneurons (transmitting impulses from the brain and spinal cord to the muscles and glands) and sensory neurons (transmitting impulses from sensory receptors along their axons toward the spinal cord and brain).

Neuropeptide: À family of transmitter substances, many of which are still being discovered, the neuropeptides are small proteins (strings of amino acids)—much larger molecules than the neurotransmitters studied earlier. Acting in the brain, neuropeptides influence emotions. Throughout the body, they act as hormones and can provide activation or suppression in the immune system (some immune cells have specific receptors on their surfaces for neuropeptides produced in the brain). The neuropeptide enkephalin is the body's natural pain killer, producing pain relief and euphoria. Another neuropeptide, substance P, is one substance involved in carrying the message of pain to the brain.

Neurotransmitter: Although nerve impulses travel electrically, the passage of impulses between neurons, or from a neuron to a muscle or glandular cell, occurs chemically. These chemicals are neurotransmitters and include the family called neuropeptides. Many neurotransmitters are identical or similar to the body's hormones.

Acting as chemical messengers, these hormone-like neurotransmitters enter the bloodstream to act at distant sites rather than within the brain itself.

Neurotransmitters and neuropeptides can affect functions and mental states as diverse as mood, memory, sensitivity to pain, sleepiness, aggression, and appetite.

When an electrical impulse travels from the nerve cell body down the axon and reaches the axon terminal, it triggers release of a neurotransmitter from swellings called synaptic knobs. The neurotransmitter crosses the synaptic gap (a billionth of an inch wide) to the dendrites of the target cell, where it binds to protein receptors.

> This opens certain receptor channels that allow sodium ions to rush into the target cell and potassium ions to leave. The flow of ions excites an area of the target cell membrane and generates an electrical impulse in the target cell. (Poole, 1986, p. 301)

Neural Plasticity: This term describes the amazing flexibility of neuronal networks to adapt to their internal and external environments. A single neuron may produce more than one kind of neurotransmitter; some neurotransmitters can act subtly by modifying the effects of other neurotransmitters; each neurotransmitter may have several types of receptor sites (serotonin has 15 currently identified); post-synaptic cells can even change the number of receptors on their surface membrane to adjust to an oversupply or deficit in a certain neurotransmitter.

Neurons can not only change the characteristics of their membranes, but they can also strengthen their synaptic connections and increase the number of connections. The process of long-term potentiation (LTP), or memory encoding, is a form of neural plasticity that occurs in the hippocampus and the neocortex. During LTP, the neurotransmitter nitric oxide (NO) acts to increase synaptic strength and convergence (the ability of a neuron to establish stronger connections with fewer target cells).

Neuromodulator: Whereas neurotransmitters directly transfer information in neural structures by activating protein receptors with ion channels, neuromodulators also activate receptors, but they exert their effect primarily indirectly by activating "second messenger pathways." Neuromodulators are substances that "appear to alter the processing characteristics of cortical structures through influences on physiological phenomenon such as synaptic transmission and pyramidal cell adaptation" (Goldstein, 1996, p. 150).

NEUROCHEMICAL LEVELS
IN NEUROSOMATIC DISORDERS

Now we will introduce the neurotransmitters, neuropeptides, and neuromodulators that are essential to an understanding of the complex chemical orchestration that is CFS/FMS.

This information appears in three parts. First, a description of the neurochemical and its role in the body. Second, its suspected dysregulation in CFS and FMS. Third, any drugs and their mode of action that Dr. Goldstein has found to correct the dysfunction. All drug names appear in italics.

Many of these neurochemicals appear in either abnormally high or low concentrations in the cerebrospinal fluid of CFS and/or FMS patients. This table provides a quick reference.

Low Levels	High Levels
Corticotropin-releasing hormone (CRH)	Substance P (SP)
Dopamine (DA)	Endothelin (ET)
Growth Hormone (GH)	
Glutamate (GT)	
Neuropeptide Y (NPY)	
Nitric Oxide (NO)	
Norepinephrine (NE)	
Oxytocin (OXT)	
Serotonin (may be low in some patients due to depression)	
Vasopressin (VP) (normal or low)	

NEUROCHEMICAL INTERRELATIONSHIPS

Many of the neurochemicals referenced in this section have relationships with one another, such as one increases or inhibits the secretion of another, or they occur in inverse proportions. This table may help you, visually, to understand the information that follows.

CO	→GT
CRH	→NE
DA	→GH
GT	→OXT
HIS	→ACh
IL–1b	→DA
IL–1b	→HIS
IL–1b	→NE
IL–1b	→SP
NE	→GH
NO	→CRH (possible)
NO	→ DA
NO	→GT
NO	→NE
NO	→Serotonin
NO	→VIP
OXT	→CRH
OXT	→NO
Serotonin	→GH
VIP	→NO

GABA$_A$	X GT	
HIS	X IL–1b	
SP	X CRH	
ATP	<–>	Adenosine
NE	<–>	SP
NPY	<–>	CRH
CRH	R	ACTH
IL–1b	R	CRH
GT	R	DA
GT	R	NE

Key: → Increases secretion or release of
      <–> Inverse relationship; when one is up, the other is down
      X   Inhibits secretion or release of
      R   Regulates

Acetylcholine (ACh)

Normal Function–ACh comes from the B-vitamin choline. ACh is the neurotransmitter released at all nerve muscle junctions that make muscles contract. ACh also provides vital neuronal communication between the brain and spinal cord. Depletion of neurons in the brain that release ACh may play a part in Alzheimer's disease. ACh exerts "cholinergic action."

The parasympathetic nervous system (see Glossary for autonomic nervous system) releases acetylcholine from its nerve endings. The PNS contains one chain of nerves passing from the brain and another from the lower spinal cord. The PNS provides the "brake" for the cardiovascular system after the sympathetic nervous system (SNS) has initiated the fight-or-flight response. The PNS releases ACh, causing blood vessels to dilate, blood pressure to drop, and heart rate to slow. The PNS dominates during sleep, slowing the heart rate and breathing, diverting blood flow to the digestive tract, and stimulating digestive organs to produce waste products. ACh also aids in maintaining sexual arousal. ACh has the opposite effects of norepinephrine and epinephrine released from the SNS.

Histamine (HIS) may increase acetylcholine secretion by modulating activity in the hippocampus and hypothalamus.

Dysfunction in CFS/FMS–Although ACh levels are normal in CFS/FMS, drugs that increase ACh may facilitate the release of neurotransmitters and increase the efficiency of synaptic transmissions.

Drug Remediation–*Nimodipine* and *ranitidine* both stimulate the release of central ACh.

Tacrine is a centrally acting cholinesterase inhibitor that increases the levels of ACh in the brain. *Tacrine* is a potassium channel blocker, and it also blocks voltage-gated sodium and calcium channels. The function of potassium channels in neurosomatic disorders is still unclear, but they do modulate cellular excitability. K channel blockers act by keeping potassium confined to intracellular regions, depolarizing cell membranes, increasing "membrane potential" to excite the cell, and stimulating the release of neurotransmitters. *Tacrine* also blocks NMDA receptor channels in the *open* state, perhaps enhancing the effect of glutamate acting at the NMDA receptor or allowing calcium ions to flow through the channel enhancing synaptic transmission. In rat studies, *tacrine* enhances NO synthase activity in the hippocampus–a finding that may be relevant to humans, given the role of NO in mediating the NMDA receptor to enhance synaptic transmission for long-term potentiation. See section on GLUTAMATE for more information about this process.

Pyridostigmine stimulates the release of peripheral ACh.

Adenosine

Normal Function–Depleted levels of brain glycogen occurring progressively during waking trigger the release of the inhibitory neurotransmitter adenosine. Stimulation of adenosine receptors then produces thalamocortical messages of an increased need for sleep. The amount of adenosine released correlates with the need for sleep. The quantity of adenosine released during non-REM sleep determines the duration and intensity of restorative, slow-wave sleep (SWS).

Adenosine levels occur in inverse proportion to levels of ATP, a potassium channel blocker. When adenosine is high and ATP is low, cells become "hyperpolarized," i.e., they are less excitable due to increased potassium conductance. The release of adenosine during sleep increases the arousal threshold, allowing uninterrupted sleep by inhibiting the effects of excitatory neurotransmitters such as acetylcholine.

Dysfunction in CFS/FMS–Disruption in the manufacture of adenosine could cause the sleep disturbances so common in neurosomatic disorders: difficulty falling asleep, light and frequently interrupted sleep, lack of restorative sleep, etc. Without enough adenosine to block excitatory neuromodulators like substance P, symptoms such as night sweats, teeth grinding, panic attacks, and nightmares could occur.

Adrenocorticotropic Hormone (ACTH)

Normal Function–Also known simply as corticotropin, adrenocorticotropic hormone (ACTH) is a neuropeptide produced by the pituitary gland that stimulates the adrenal cortex (the outer layer of the adrenal glands) to release corticosteroid hormones, including hydrocortisone (cortisol). Levels of ACTH increase with injury, infection, burns, surgery, stress, emotion, and decreased blood pressure.

Dysfunction in CFS/FMS–ACTH occurs at normal levels in CFS/FMS patients, but it does increase secretion of endothelin, already found in excess in CFS/FMS patients. Excess endothelin, a vaso-constrictor, may explain the baseline reduced rCBF in CFS/FMS patients. Endothelin also induces the secretion of substance P and causes hypermetabolic activity in the brain.

Carbon Monoxide (CO)

Normal Function–Both carbon monoxide (CO) and nitric oxide (NO) are retrograde neurotransmitters involved in long-term potentiation, or memory encoding, in the hippocampus and neocortex. CO acts in the same fashion as NO to enhance synaptic strength through increasing glutamate secretion at the presynaptic neuron. CO may also be important in stimulating the secretion of corticotropin-releasing hormone (CRH).

Dysfunction in CFS/FMS–A CO deficiency may partially account for low levels of CRH in CFS. This, along with the NO deficiency could impair the process of memory encoding in CFS patients.

Corticotropin-Releasing Hormone (CRH)

Normal Function–Corticotropin-releasing hormone (CRH) is a neuropeptide secreted by an area of the hypothalamus called the paraventricular nucleus (PVN). CRH regulates the secretion of ACTH, and hence cortisol, as well as other substances. CRH also helps regulate the prefrontal cortex (PFC), the locus ceruleus (LC), and the sympathetic nervous system (see Glossary for autonomic nervous system). CRH is immunosuppressive, stimulating the secretion of cortisol (hydrocortisone) to reduce inflammation and producing sympathetic activity in the spleen and lymphatic organs.

Both the PFC and LC contain receptors for CRH. CRH increases PFC norepinephrine (NE), either by acting on the LC to produce NE or on presynaptic neurons in the PFC itself–perhaps both.

CRH appears to be the mediator of core body temperature after exercise, rather than the heat generated by the exercise itself. Core temperature rises with a change in the thermoregulatory set-point, controlled by the hypothalamus and mediated by CRH.

Dysfunction in CFS/FMS—Levels are low, possibly due to high levels of substance P, which inhibits CRH, or by an antagonist to IL-1 beta, which regulates CRH. Since CRH is immunosuppressive, reduced levels could cause activation of the immune system as in CFS (fever, swollen lymph nodes, sore throat, etc.). In exercise stress studies of IL-1 regulated functions, "we failed to find the expected increases in cortisol, IL-1, IL-6, catecholamines, growth hormone, beta-endorphin, somatostatin, and core body temperature after exercise" (Goldstein, 1996, p. 23). These unexpectedly low hormone levels and unchanged or lowered core body temperatures point to a malfunction in neurohormonal mediation by CRH and the hypothalamus itself, which maintains the body's temperature set-point. A mechanism similar to this may be responsible for the temperature intolerance common among CFS/FMS patients.

Low levels of CRH also lead to low levels of norepinephrine (NE), due to CRH's role in regulating the PFC and the LC. NE increases the signal-to-noise (STN) ratio, and low levels of NE impair the ability to screen out irrelevant stimuli.

CRH deficiency can also result in sleepiness, a common neurosomatic complaint.

Brain structures appear in rectangles; neurochemicals in ellipses.

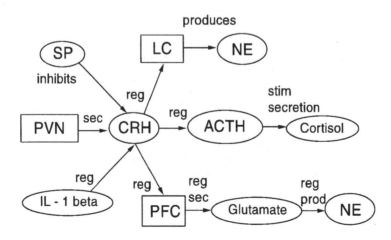

Drug Remediation–Mexiletine may act by increasing the secretion of central CRH. *Lidocaine*, known best as a local anesthetic, when given intravenously, will act in the hypothalamus to increase secretion of central CRH. *Lidocaine*, when it acts as an analgesic, increases cerebral blood flow. When it acts to rapidly relieve global CFS/FMS symptoms, it decreases cerebral blood flow, as do all other successful agents. This may be more a result of the increase in NE (a vasoconstrictor) that accompanies an increase in central CRH.

Ranitidine increases central CRH by inhibiting suppression of IL-1 beta, which regulates CRH.

Oxytocin stimulates the secretion of peripheral CRH.

Dopamine (DA)

Normal Function–Concentrated in the brainstem, neurons containing the neurotransmitter dopamine (DA) connect with the limbic system and the frontal lobes. Too much DA in the frontal lobes can cause symptoms of schizophrenia. Through different connections, dopamine-containing neurons reach the basal ganglia, which orchestrate complex movements. Low levels of dopamine can cause motor problems, and at the extreme, Parkinson's disease.

Dopamine reduces fatigue, enhances cognition, stimulates behavior, and regulates mood and activity.

Dopamine pathways predominate in the left hemisphere of the cerebral cortex, which specializes in cognitive routines.

Dysfunction in CFS/FMS–DA occurs in low levels in CFS/FMS patients, possibly due to decreased glutamate secretion from the prefrontal cortex (the PFC secretes glutamate that then regulates production of norepinephrine and dopamine).

Higher concentrations of dopamine in certain parts of the brain are indicative of stress tolerance. Susceptibility to stress in CFS/FMS patients is consistent with low levels of dopamine.

The metabolites of dopamine, norepinephrine, and serotonin (5-HIAA), all of which are low in the CSF of FMS patients, are believed to stimulate the release of growth hormone (GH). GH is essential for the ongoing process of muscle maintenance and repair. Not only is GH low, but the products induced by its secretion are also low (Bennett and Russell, 1993).

DA deficiency can also result in sleepiness, a common neurosomatic complaint.

Drug Remediation–All antidepressants may provide relief for CFS/FMS sufferers by increasing extracellular dopamine in the prefrontal cortex.

Nimodipine causes a release of dopamine.

Venlafaxine blocks reuptake of dopamine.

Risperidone may enhance midbrain release of dopamine.

Pyridostigmine may induce the adrenal glands to produce more catecholamines (including norepinephrine and dopamine).

Endothelin (ET)

Normal Function–The neuropeptide endothelin (ET) is the most powerful vasoconstrictor in the body. Endothelin increases cerebral metabolism while it decreases cerebral blood flow–the opposite of what one would expect since increased metabolism demands more blood. Endothelin results in increased secretion of glutamate, dopamine, and nitric oxide.

Endothelin receptors reside in neuronal, neuroendocrine, and endocrine cells as well as in endothelial cells (a layer of cells lining the heart, blood vessels, and ducts of the lymphatic system). Endothelin receptors are present in high density in the hypothalamus and the rest of the limbic system. Endothelins play a role in long-term cellular regulation but may also participate in certain stress related disorders, including depression.

NO produced by endothelial cells is involved in the process of long-term potentiation (LTP) in the hippocampus and neocortex.

Dysfunction in CFS/FMS–The cerebrospinal fluid of FMS patients contains elevated levels of endothelin. Excess endothelin may account for the baseline cerebral hypoperfusion found in CFS/FMS patients due to its vasoconstrictor properties. Excess endothelin induces the secretion of substance P, which has the effect of widening receptive fields, helping to explain the bodywide pain of FMS. With an excess of endothelin, hypermetabolic (increased metabolic) activity occurs in the brain. Increased metabolism demands more blood, but endothelin's vasoconstrictor properties prevent additional blood from entering the brain.

With exercise and cognitive activities placing additional demands on cerebral metabolism, endothelin may further reduce rCBF in CFS/FMS patients.

Drug Remediation–The high number of receptors for endothelin in the hypothalamus and other parts of the limbic system provides a route for drugs that will bind to endothelin receptors, and consequently produce lower endothelin levels.

Nimodipine, an L-type calcium channel blocker (see Glossary for calcium channel blockers), controls the hypermetabolic activity associated with excess endothelin.

Excess endothelin causes an increase in dopamine stimulation. Calcium channel blockers and *hydralazine* will lessen dopamine secretion.

Gamma-Amino Butyric Acid (GABA)

Normal Function–Gamma-amino butyric acid (GABA) is a neurotransmitter that controls the transmission of nerve impulses by blocking the release of certain other neurotransmitters, such as norepinephrine and dopamine, that stimulate nerve activity.

The inhibitory action of GABA in the thalamus and the ventromedial nucleus of the hypothalamus (VMH) is of most interest in neurosomatic disorders.

GABA is particularly important in regulating restorative, slow-wave sleep (SWS).

Dysfunction in CFS/FMS–Messages regarding touch and pain travel to the thalamus by separate routes, but they travel together from there to the cortex. They can do this because of the inhibitory nature of GABA: When pain is the sensation, GABA inhibits messages regarding touch. Impaired GABA secretion from the thalamic reticular nuclei can cause both touch and actual pain to register as pain. This could be a mechanism to explain the central pain component of FMS.

In the VMH, the $GABA_A$ system works to inhibit the release of glutamate, slowing energy metabolism.

Reduced secretion of GABA could result in interruption of SWS due to its inhibitory action toward excitatory neurotransmitters.

Drug Remediation–Drugs that enhance the effect of GABA, such as *alprazolam*, or those that mimic the effect of GABA, such as *gabapentin* and *lamotrigine*, act in the thalamus to reduce centrally mediated pain.

Baclofen is a $GABA_B$ agonist. Symptomatically, *baclofen* is most effective in reducing central pain (FMS, headache, low back pain, etc.). It is also effective in providing supraspinal analgesia (i.e., centrally above the spinal cord), suppressing panic attacks, reducing cacosmia (odor hypersensitivity), reducing multiple chemical sensitivity, reducing anxiety, and increasing alertness. From a neurochemical standpoint, *baclofen* inhibits CRH release, stimulates GH release, which in turn increases insulin-like growth factor-1; and inhibits the release of dopamine.

Felbamate enhances the function of $GABA_A$ receptors when there is a reduction in GABA neurotransmission. *Felbamate* may work synergistically with *gabapentin* in CFS/FMS patients.

Gabapentin (GBP) acts to increase the available pool of GABA in the central nervous system and may enhance the functioning of the thalamic reticular nucleus. Symptomatically, GBP increases energy and reduces anxiety. Neurochemically, GBP increases GABA, inhibiting an inhibitory system in the thalamic reticular nucleus (RT), resulting in thalamocortical excitation.

Lidocaine is a GABA reuptake inhibitor.

Glutamate (GT)

Normal Function–The prefrontal cortex (PFC) projects excitatory neurons that secrete the excitatory amino acid glutamate (GT) to brainstem nuclei, causing the production of "biogenic amines," particularly dopamine (DA) and norepinephrine (NE).

Nitric oxide (NO) and carbon monoxide (CO) both induce the secretion of GT. Post-synaptic neurons secrete NO and CO, which diffuse in a retrograde manner back into the presynaptic neuron (which is already firing and releasing a neurotransmitter), inducing it to release glutamate. Secretion of glutamate activates the N-methyl-D-aspartate (NMDA) receptor, depolarizing post-synaptic receptor sites (i.e., causing magnesium ions that are blocking NMDA receptor sites to leave) and allowing calcium ions to flow through NMDA receptor channels, enhancing synaptic transmission.

This is especially important in the process of long-term potentiation, involved in memory encoding, which occurs in the hippocampus and neocortex.

Brain structures appear in rectangles; neurochemicals in ellipses.

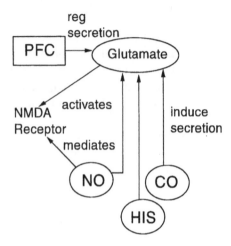

*Dysfunction in CFS/FMS–*There is a reduction in glutamate secretion from the prefrontal cortex (the PFC secretes glutamate, which then regulates production of norepinephrine and dopamine).

GT may also be deficient in the DLPFC of CFS patients.

Impaired ability to form new memories in CFS relates to weakened synaptic convergence in the hippocampus and neocortex. This is primarily an impairment in presynaptic glutamate secretion that results in not clearing the magnesium ion blocks on post-synaptic NMDA receptor sites to allow calcium ions to flow, which potentiates synaptic transmission enhanced by NO.

GT deficiency can also result in sleepiness, a common neurosomatic complaint.

*Drug Remediation–*The process of memory encoding can theoretically be gated by controlling either presynaptic glutamate secretion or post-synaptic retrograde neurotransmitter production of CO or NO in encoding areas within the hippocampus and neocortex.

Cycloserine enhances glutamate transmission.

Glycine is a drug as well as an inhibitory neurotransmitter within the brainstem and spinal cord. Glycine acts to enhance glutamate transmission in its role as an "obligatory co-agonist" at the NMDA channel. Unless glycine occupies its site on the NMDA receptor, the NMDA channel will not open for glutamate.

Growth Hormone (GH)

Normal Function–The pituitary gland secretes the growth hormone (GH), or somatotropin, the main regulator of height. It stimulates the growth of bone and muscle, maintains cellular rates of protein synthesis, and speeds the breakdown of fats used as energy for growth. The neuronal systems involved in the onset and maintenance of sleep also trigger neuroendocrine responses during slow-wave sleep (SWS), most importantly, the release of growth hormone.

Dysfunction in CFS/FMS–Levels of growth hormone are deficient in FMS patients. The body needs GH to repair the daily occurrences of muscle microtrauma (small breaks in muscle cell membranes caused from overuse). GH levels tend to peak in the body between midnight and 2 a.m., a period of often disturbed sleep in FMS patients (Bennett, 1995).

Reduced secretion of GH may result from alpha-wave intrusion into SWS, or functional abnormalities in the caudate nucleus of the basal ganglia or the orbitofrontal cortex (the anatomical areas associated with producing SWS).

Drug Remediation–*Pyridostigmine*, while not crossing the blood-brain barrier, still increases secretion of GH. It also increases secretion of growth hormone-releasing hormone, perhaps by its stimulation of the superior cervical ganglion (SCG).

Sumatriptan, commonly employed to stop migraine headaches, increases the release of growth hormone in neurosomatic patients.

Baclofen also stimulates the release of GH.

Histamine (HIS)

Normal Function–An excitatory neurotransmitter residing on cells throughout the body, histamine release occurs during an allergic reaction and causes inflammation. Histamine (HIS) also stimulates production of stomach acid and narrows the bronchi (airways) in the lungs.

While histamine suppresses IL-1 beta, IL-1 beta stimulates the central release of histamine, a process that results in elevating body temperature.

HIS enhances NMDA-mediated synaptic transmission in the hippo-campus and neocortex, where it could improve the process of long-term potentiation (LTP). This is consistent with studies in rats which have indicated that depletion of histamine decreases memory and learning.

HIS also occurs in the superior cervical ganglion (SCG) of rats. The SCG comprise part of the autonomic nervous system.

The basal ganglia and structures of the limbic system contain large numbers of type-2 histamine receptors (H_2 receptors). Hista-mine may be responsible for increasing acetylcholine secretion by modulating activity in the hippocampus and hypothalamus.

Histamine may play a role in sleep-wake cycles and circadian rhythms by inducing melatonin secretion.

Dysfunction in CFS/FMS–Histamine levels are normal in CFS/FMS patients.

Drug Remediation–Ranitidine is an antagonist at the H_2 receptor site. H_2 blockers are cholinesterase inhibitors and exert a central cho-linergic effect (i.e., they increase brain ACh). Increasing ACh, the neurotransmitter of the PNS, causes the SNS to counterbalance its effects by increasing NE neurotransmission. This may explain how the H_2 blocker *ranitidine* can work in the SCG to increase central NE.

By blocking histamine release from H_2 receptors in the hypothal-amus, *ranitidine* may also inhibit the suppression of IL-1 beta. Increased levels of IL-I beta would then result in increased levels of the immunosuppressive CRH (IL-1 beta regulates CRH), account-ing for relief from CFS symptoms of overactive immune response, such as low-grade fever, sore throat, and swollen glands.

Interleukin-1 (IL-1)

Normal Function–Macrophages, the scavengers of the immune system, produce IL-1 beta when they encounter a foreign organism. The IL-1 travels to a cluster of neurons within the hypothalamus where it prompts the temperature regulator to set a higher tempera-ture. The body then starts to conserve heat by constricting blood vessels in the skin to prevent heat loss and causes the muscles to contract, producing shivering. IL-1 also breaks down stored fats to warm the body. The increased body temperature enhances the effi-ciency of the body's infection-fighting agents.

IL-1 beta regulates secretion of CRH, stimulates the secretion of substance P, and may stimulate the secretion of biogenic amines (norepinephrine and dopamine) directly, without concurrent elevation of CRH levels.

While histamine suppresses IL-1 beta, IL-1 beta stimulates the central release of histamine, a process that results in elevating body temperature.

IL-1 beta increases sleepiness.

Dysfunction in CFS/FMS–Through its regulation of CRH secretion–and hence cortisol release–IL-1 beta influences the immune response. With a reduction in CRH levels comes a reduction in its immunosuppressive effects. This leaves the immune system activated, accounting for CFS symptoms such as low-grade fever, sore throat, and swelling of lymph nodes.

Since IL-1 beta levels are normal in CFS/FMS patients and since IL-1 beta regulates secretion of CRH, one would expect CRH levels to be normal also. The fact that CRH levels are low has led Dr. Goldstein to postulate that an antagonist mechanism is interfering with the activity of IL-1 beta.

IL-1 beta also stimulates the secretion of substance P. Normal IL-1 beta levels leave elevated levels of substance P in FMS patients unexplained, however. High substance P levels are also inconsistent with the theory of an antagonist mechanism that might reduce the effects of IL-1 beta. Perhaps another explanation for elevated substance P levels would be competition for nerve growth factor (see section on substance P).

Neuropeptide Y (NPY)

Normal Function–Neuropeptide Y (NPY) is the neuropeptide occurring in the greatest concentrations within the brain. NPY is a powerful vasoconstrictor, released primarily in the limbic system and cerebral cortex. It reduces anxiety and can stimulate appetite and cause weight gain. NPY occurs in inverse proportion to CRH, the immunosuppressive neuropeptide that releases cortisol. Under certain conditions, NPY releases NO or occurs in conjunction with it.

Dysfunction in CFS/FMS–NPY likely occurs at reduced levels in CFS/FMS patients. This could result from its co-localization with NE, also reduced as a result of decreased levels of glutamate.

Any dysregulation in NPY secretion could lead to disruption of circadian rhythms and could explain some of the sleep disturbance problems associated with neurosomatic disorders.

Drug Remediation–Because of the inverse relationship between NPY and CRH, drug therapies that might attempt to raise NPY would then lower CRH, which is already low in CFS/FMS patients. Therefore, such therapies would be counterproductive.

The vasoconstrictor properties of NPY (along with NE) may make it one of the primary players in the reduced cerebral blood flow observed after administration of one of Dr. Goldstein's rapidly acting, successful CFS/FMS drug treatments.

Sumatriptan, commonly employed to stop migraine headaches, causes a three-fold increase in NPY in neurosomatic patients.

Nitric Oxide (NO)

Normal Function–Nitric oxide (NO) is a gaseous neurotransmitter and the primary vasodilator in the brain. NO is believed to regulate local blood flow, to signal the release of other neurotransmitters, and to regulate synaptic efficiency.

NO synthase (the enzyme that acts on arginine to manufacture NO) occurs in concentrated levels in the hippocampus and other sites of sensory gating.

Role of NO in Regulating Synaptic Efficiency

NO, secreted by endothelial cells, acts in the hippocampus and neocortex as a "retrograde neurotransmitter" to enhance the presynaptic activity of neurons involved in long-term potentiation, or memory encoding. NO is secreted from the post-synaptic neuron and then diffuses back (i.e., in a retrograde fashion) into the firing, presynaptic neuron that is already releasing its neurotransmitter. At the presynaptic neuron, NO stimulates glutamate secretion, which "potentiates" the synaptic connection, allowing a stronger signal to pass. NO may also increase "synaptic convergence," a process by which an individual neuron makes stronger connections with fewer target cells.

Relationship with IL-1 Beta

IL-1 beta can stimulate the production of NO synthase (the first step in the production of NO). Levels of NO may be indirectly determined by the level of citrulline, the end product of NO's manufacture, in the cerebrospinal fluid. In CFS/FMS patients, citrulline is low. One might expect low levels of IL-1 beta to accompany low levels of NO, but this is not the case: IL-1 beta levels are normal in the CSF of CFS/FMS patients. Since production of IL-1 beta seems normal, perhaps something is inhibiting the action of IL-1 beta that is, in turn, inhibiting NO synthase.

Relationship with IL-1 Beta and Sleep

Whatever the mechanism causing low levels of NO, it could also have the effect of reducing central nervous system levels of serotonin, dopamine, CRH, and other substances. The interleukins are crucial to the process of serotonin synthesis, and IL-1 and IL-1 beta are both known to induce sleepiness themselves. Inhibited NO synthesis in rats diminishes the amount and duration of their non-REM sleep. NO is therefore assumed to have a role in maintaining spontaneous sleep, and may act as the "sleep coordinator" for several sleep factors.

Relationship with the N-Methyl-D-Aspartate (NMDA) Receptor

NO stimulates the secretion of glutamate (GT) and mediates the action of the NMDA receptor, one of glutamate's major sites of action. NMDA receptor sites in the spinal cord are active during the processing of nociceptive information, making NO a key modulator for peripheral pain processing and sensory gating.

NO releases dopamine and inhibits its uptake (making more available). It also stimulates the release of serotonin and norepinephrine.

NO stimulates the secretion of vasointestinal peptide (VIP), and vice versa. VIP is crucial for neuronal survival.

Dysfunction in CFS/FMS–There is a central deficiency of NO, and NO is essential for efficient processing in neuronal assemblies.

The difficulty CFS/FMS patients have with short-term memory may be the result of decreased levels of NO in the hippocampus and the neocortex that weaken long-term potentiation by decreasing synaptic strength and convergence.

Sensory gating abnormalities in CFS/FMS probably relate to low levels of NO. NO plays a role in processing peripheral nociceptive information.

NO is anxiolytic, or anxiety reducing. Low levels of NO could be contributing to the concomitant anxiety usually found in CFS/FMS patients.

Low levels of dopamine in CFS/FMS patients may be due to low levels of NO. Reduced dopamine can cause fatigue, impair cognition, lessen attention, and depress behavior.

Low levels of NO could contribute to sleep disorders in CFS/FMS, given NO's role in maintaining spontaneous sleep.

Drug Remediation–Nitroglycerin converts to NO and normally elicits a vasodilatory effect. However, when it relieves the symptoms of CFS/FMS, it causes further cerebral vasoconstriction, or reduced rCBF, as do all other rapidly acting, successful agents.

The process of memory encoding can theoretically be gated by controlling either presynaptic glutamate secretion, or post-synaptic retrograde neurotransmitter production of CO or NO in encoding areas within the hippocampus and neocortex. The drug *oxytocin* appears to do the latter by increasing levels of NO. As with all other rapidly acting, successful agents, it also causes increased global cerebral hypoperfusion.

Norepinephrine (NE)

*Normal Function–*Concentrated in the brainstem, neurons containing the neurotransmitter norepinephrine (NE) are active during the waking state, particularly during emotional arousal. Since we learn most efficiently when emotionally involved, NE may be important in memory encoding. Depression can occur with low levels of NE and a related neurotransmitter, serotonin. NE influences such diverse functions as sleep, memory, and stress reactions, and emotional states such as aggressiveness, pleasure, and rage.

Nerve endings of the sympathetic nervous system (SNS) release norepinephrine and epinephrine. The SNS consists of two chains of nerves passing from the spinal cord to the organs and other structures of the body they control. NE's primary purpose is to maintain blood pressure by stimulating the constriction of certain vessels when blood pressure drops below normal. These neurotransmitters prepare the body for action and are active in the fight-or-flight response to danger or perceived danger. They increase heart rate, widen airways, bring blood into the muscles, constrict blood vessels in the skin and abdomen in order to increase blood to the muscles, slow down the digestive system, dilate the pupils, and are involved in orgasm. In addition to being produced by neurons, the adrenal glands also secrete NE.

Norepinephrine is paramount in the processing of sensory input due to its role in enhancing the signal-to-noise (STN) ratio. A high STN ratio allows the organism to screen out irrelevant stimuli and to accurately perceive and process input of survival value.

Norepinephrine pathways predominate to the right hemisphere of the cerebral cortex, which specializes in novel cognitive situations.

Dysfunction in CFS/FMS–NE occurs in low levels in CFS/FMS patients, possibly due to decreased glutamate secretion from the prefrontal cortex (the PFC secretes glutamate that then regulates production of norepinephrine and dopamine). Events that trigger or worsen CFS/FMS–such as infection, inhalation of anesthesia, immunization, focusing attention, or exercise–deplete the brain's store of NE.

Functional problems will occur in the involuntary processes of the autonomic nervous system without enough NE and may result in dysautonomia, the symptoms of which include fluctuating low blood pressure, Raynaud's phenomenon, thermoregulatory dysfunction, and rapid heart rate, among others.

The fragile encoding of memories found in CFS patients may be attributable to low levels of NE and the resulting inadequate filtering of irrelevant stimuli by the noradrenergic (NE producing) fibers of the locus ceruleus. The resulting low signal-to-noise (STN) ratio accounts for the complaint among CFS patients of feeling bombarded with input and being easily distracted and unable to focus.

The metabolites of norepinephrine, dopamine, and serotonin (5-HIAA), all of which are low in the CSF of FMS patients, are believed to stimulate the release of growth hormone (GH). GH is essential for the ongoing process of muscle maintenance and repair. Not only is GH low, but the products induced by its secretion are also low (Bennett and Russell, 1993).

NE deficiency can also result in sleepiness, a common neurosomatic complaint.

Drug Remediation–Naphazoline HC1, nitroglycerin, nimodipine, hydralazine, pyridostigmine, mexiletine, and *lidocaine* probably all cause further reduction of rCBF by stimulating the release of norepinephrine (NE) with subsequent enhanced secretion of corticotropin releasing hormone (CRH). *Lidocaine,* mexiletine, and *naphazoline* HCl also decrease secretion of substance P (SP).

The vasoconstrictor properties of NE (along with NPY, which is longer acting) may make it one of the primary players in the reduced cerebral blood flow observed after administration of one of Dr. Goldstein's rapidly acting, successful CFS/FMS drug treatments.

Venlafaxine, desipramine, and *lidocaine* are all NE reuptake inhibitors.

Pyridostigmine may induce the adrenal glands to produce more catecholamines (including norepinephrine and dopamine).

Nefazodone, pindolol, and *risperidone* all act to increase the glutamate-evoked secretion of NE from the locus ceruleus.

Oxytocin (OXT)

*Normal Function–*Oxytocin (OXT) is a neuropeptide hormone produced by the pituitary gland that causes uterine contractions during labor and stimulates lactation in nursing mothers.

> OXT neurons project to many areas of the limbic system and brainstem, as well as to the frontal cortex. Brain OXT is involved in organization of maternal behavior, female and male sexual behavior, feeding, social behavior, and memory. OXT also has effects on cardiovascular (as an arterial vasoconstrictor), autonomic, and thermoregulatory processes (Goldstein, 1996, p. 156).

OXT is also active in the stress response and has a pronounced effect on libido, increasing arousal in both sexes.

"OXT neurons may be the main source of nitric oxide (NO) production in the hypothalamic-pituitary system" (Goldstein, 1996). There are two areas of the hypothalamus with OXT-secreting neurons. Both areas also secrete vasopressin (VP) and corticotropin-releasing hormone (CRH).

OXT may be important in modulating the function of the hippocampus.

Both glutamatergic (glutamate producing) and catecholaminergic (amine producing, for example, norepinephrine and dopamine) neurons in the brainstem stimulate OXT secretion from the paraventricular nucleus of the hypothalamus (PVN).

Dysfunction in CFS/FMS–OXT levels may be low in CFS. Since OXT induces the secretion of CRH, this may help to explain low CRH levels in CFS/FMS patients.

The food intolerance experienced by many neurosomatic patients could relate to the function of OXT in mediating afferent (stomach to brain) sensory input and dysregulated gating of that input by the PFC.

Drug Remediation–Oxytocin, available under the trade name Pitocin, is administered by intramuscular injection. Symptomatically, it improves cognition, reduces the pain of FMS, increases libido, reduces anxiety, and reduces depression. OXT is present in sympathetic ganglia where it must exert its effect because of its inability to pass the blood-brain barrier and its short half-life in the body.

OXT probably acts through modulation of brain monoaminergic transmission. Monoaminergic refers to the liberation or involvement of monoamines, such as serotonin and norepinephrine.

Serotonin (5-HT)

Normal Function–A neurotransmitter in the brain involved in controlling states of consciousness (such as sleep and waking) and mood. Low levels of both serotonin and norepinephrine can result in depression. The substance serotonin is also present in other parts of the body where it slows bleeding by constricting small blood vessels and in the digestive tract where it inhibits secretion of gastric fluids and stimulates smooth muscle action in the intestines. At elevated levels, serotonin will diminish sensitivity to pain, decrease carbohydrate craving, and induce sleep.

Serotonin (5-HT), "has been implicated in controlling feeding behavior, thermoregulation, sexual behavior, sleep, and pain modulation" (Goldstein, 1996, p. 105).

5-HT is particularly important in the onset of restorative, slow-wave sleep (SWS). Serotonin-containing neurons also act to dampen sensory input and to decrease motor activity at the onset of sleep.

Dysfunction in CFS/FMS–Central serotonin levels in the CSF of CFS/FMS patients have been somewhat low in one study, and normal in another. Low levels in some patients may represent those CFS/FMS patients who also suffer from depression.

The fact that obsessive-compulsive disorders (OCDs) respond to serotonin reuptake inhibitors, coupled with the fact that OCDs are uncommon in neurosomatic patients, leads to the premise that serotonin deficiency is not important in the pathology of neurosomatic disorders.

The metabolites of serotonin (5-HIAA), dopamine, norepinephrine, all of which are low in the CSF of FMS patients, are believed to stimulate the release of growth hormone (GH). GH is essential for the ongoing process of muscle maintenance and repair. Not only is GH low, but the products induced by its secretion are also low (Bennett and Russell, 1993).

Drug Remediation–*Nimodipine* causes release of serotonin. Serotonin, since it is vasoactive, is possibly one of the secondary messengers that contribute to the reduced rCBF produced by drugs in Dr. Goldstein's rapidly acting protocol.

Pindolol is a beta-blocker (see Glossary), as well as an antagonists at the 5-HT$_{1A}$ serotonin receptor. Serotonin lessens the glutamate-evoked activation of locus ceruleus (LC) neurons, decreasing their production of norepinephrine (NE). Therefore, a serotonin antagonist like *pindolol* would result in increasing glutamate-evoked NE secretion, to the benefit of neurosomatic patients. The use of *pindolol* along with serotonin reuptake inhibitors (SRIs) seems to augment the antidepressant effect of the SRIs by permitting the release of more serotonin.

Doxepin, venlafaxine, and *nefazodone* are all serotonin reuptake inhibitors.

Risperidone and *nefazodone* are both antagonists at the 5-HT$_2$ serotonin receptor.

The serotonin 5-HT$_2$ receptor is important in neurosomatic disorders for a number of reasons:

- 5-HT$_2$ receptor sites are found in the cortex, caudate nucleus of the basal ganglia, limbic system, midbrain, and hypothalamus–all areas believed to be dysfunctional in CFS/FMS. Antagonists at the 5-HT_2 receptor may enhance dopamine (DA) release from midbrain sites (DA levels are low in CFS/FMS patients).

- The 5-HT_2 receptor is active in "vasoconstriction, migraine, anxiety, depression, and sleep" (Goldstein, 1996, p. 167). *Risperidone* increases stage 3 and stage 4 slow-wave sleep (SWS), which is often impaired in CFS/FMS patients.

- The 5-HT_2 receptor plays a role in increasing the density of glucocorticoid (GR) receptors in the hippocampus and other limbic sites. Glucocorticoids inhibit the release of corticosteroids from the adrenal glands and thus mediate the stress response. Elevated density of both GR and mineralocorticoid (MR) receptors is evident in CFS, possibly due to genetic predisposition combined with an early childhood event, altering the stress response of the individual and possibly leading to limbic system dysfunction. Antagonists at the 5-HT_2 receptor site act to decrease this GR receptor density.

  Both GR and MR receptors mediate the stress response: MR receptors in determining the sensitivity of the response (i.e., evaluation and choosing a response), and GR receptors in terminating the response (i.e., learning and memory). It is the balance between these receptors that determines an organism's ability to adaptively respond to its environment.

Sumatriptan is an agonist at the 5-HT_{1D} serotonin receptor. It probably acts there to stop the release of peptides involved in the neurogenic inflammatory response that defines a migraine headache. *Sumatriptan* may directly block trigeminal nerve transmission, and it may be a dysfunction in the neural transmission through the trigeminovascular system that causes migraines. In neurosomatic patients, *sumatriptan* causes an increase in growth hormone and a tripling of neuropeptide Y (NPY) levels. Anatomically, *sumatriptan* may alter a complex neural network comprising the trigeminal nerve, locus ceruleus, reticular formation, and dorsal raphe nucleus to decrease diffuse pain and increase the signal-to-noise ratio. Symptomatically, neurosomatic patients may experience a decrease in pain with *sumatriptan*. A lucky few may experience total amelioration of their symptoms. When it is effective in eliminating

CFS/FMS symptoms, *sumatriptan* produces global cerebral hypo-perfusion, just as all other successful agents.

Substance P (SP)

Normal Function–Substance P is the neuropeptide that transmits pain signals along peripheral nerve fibers from the pain site through the spinal cord and to the brain. In response, special neurons in the brain and spinal cord release endorphins, the body's natural pain-killers. The endorphins bind to opiate receptors on the pain-trans-mitting neurons, preventing them from firing, which in turn reduces the production of SP. Fewer pain impulses reach the brain and the individual experiences some pain relief.

NE and SP have an inverse relationship: when one is high, the other is low. SP lowers the signal-to-noise (STN) ratio, whereas NE raises it. When the STN ratio is adequately high, the organism can screen out irrelevant sensory input, allowing through only stimuli of survival value.

Dysfunction in CFS/FMS–Substance P occurs at three times the normal level in the cerebrospinal fluid (CSF) of FMS patients. Sub-stance P inhibits the release of corticotropin-releasing hormone (CRH), which is low in CFS/FMS patients. Is elevated substance P responsible for the low levels of CRH, or is there another contributing mechanism, such as an antagonist affecting the ability of IL-1 beta to regulate CRH levels?

Substance P may act as a nocturnally excitatory neuromodulator, producing night sweats, teeth grinding, nocturnal panic attacks, and nightmares. This is probably due to impaired production of adeno-sine, which, in sufficient quantity, hyperpolarizes neurons (lessens their excitability), increasing the arousal threshold and allowing quick return to sleep after transient awakenings.

Since SP lowers the STN ratio, high levels of substance P accom-panied by low levels of NE would lead to further reductions in the STN ratio, impairing the ability to filter out irrelevant stimuli. This could account for the stress CFS patients experience in environ-ments replete with sensory input; for example, when in shopping malls or on freeways, CFS patients sense that too much is coming at them at once.

Another theory of Dr. Goldstein's is that since both SP and NE compete for a substance called nerve growth factor (NGF) and because NE is low, the SP neurons have an advantage in competition for NGF over NE neurons. Thus, SP neurons increase in number, and more SP is secreted than is usual. This theory would be consistent with the finding that SP levels do not correlate with FMS pain levels.

In FMS patients, the thalamus and other areas of the brain secrete excess SP and the related neurokinin A during muscle contraction, and secretion continues even after the contraction ceases. Dysregulation in the secretion of these substances could account for the postexertional fatigue experienced by FMS patients especially if the dysregulation is not counterbalanced by increased secretion of NE.

Excess SP may be the neurochemical expression of fear and insecurity during childhood development that results in hypervigilance. SP, because it widens receptive fields, would allow the individual to process a wider array of stimuli. This is one of the developmental components that Dr. Goldstein believes may contribute to the onset of neurosomatic illnesses.

Drug Remediation–Dr. Goldstein believes that many of the drugs in his protocol that cause reduced rCBF and rapid relief of CFS/FMS symptoms do so by first releasing NE and NPY. The release of these neurotransmitters then triggers CRH secretion and SP inhibition. Inhibition of SP is probably due to its inverse relationship with NE.

Mexiletine, naphazoline, and *lidocaine* inhibit the release of substance P in mice may have relevance for humans.

Sumatriptan may block trigeminal nerve transmission of substance P.

Vasoactive Intestinal Peptide (VIP)

Normal Function–A neuropeptide that stimulates the production of nerve growth factors, nitric oxide (NO), and IL-1-alpha and beta. Both VIP and the IL-1 it induces are essential for survival of neurons. VIP also works with other substances to induce sleep.

VIP potentiates the action of glutamate in its role in maintaining circadian rhythms.

NO stimulates the secretion of VIP and is stimulated by it.

Dysfunction in CFS/FMS–VIP levels are normal in CFS/FMS patients. However, by its action of stimulating the secretion of NO, VIP plays a role in long-term potentiation, which is often impaired in CFS/FMS patients. Also, by stimulating nerve growth factors (NGF), VIP could potentially have the effect of lowering elevated substance P levels by decreasing the competition between SP and NE for NGF. SP levels may be high because NE is too low to attract enough NGF for the paramount task of nerve growth.

Drug Protocol Reference Table

Symbols are used to denote the following:

*Side effects listed are those experienced at standard therapeutic doses and may not be expected to occur until the drug has been in use for some time. Remember that Dr. Goldstein will usually try only one dose of a drug as he moves through the protocol. These are listed for your reference in the event that Dr. Goldstein prescribes the drug for you on a long-term basis.

**These drugs all cause decreased regional cerebral blood flow (rCBF), hypoperfusion, when they result in rapid and profound relief of CFS/FMS symptoms.

DRUG NAME	MARKETED FOR	MODE OF ACTION	EFFECT OF DRUG ON NEUROSOMATIC PATIENTS	POSSIBLE SIDE EFFECTS *	ONSET OF ACTION	DURATION OF ACTION
Naphazoline HCl (eye drops)	Generic decongestant Minor eye irritation	** Peripherally acting ocular alpha adrenergic agonist (increases release of norepinephrine); decreases Substance P	Decreases pain, fatigue, anxiety, and tender point sensitivity; increases cognitive clarity; can resolve multiple chemical sensitivity (MCS)	Nervousness, insomnia mild burning of eyes	2-3 sec	3-6 hrs
Nitroglycerin (sublingual tablet)	Antianginal agent; prevention/ treatment of chest pains	** Generic vasodilator; produces cerebral vasodilation by conversion to nitric oxide (NO)	Relieves pain	Headache, feeling faint, flushing rapid heart rate	2-3 min	3-6 hrs
Nimodipine	Vasodilator- for func. loss after stroke; migraine/ cluster head-ache preven-tion	** L-type calcium channel blocker; works by interfering with muscle contraction by blocking movement of calcium across muscle membranes (as muscles relax and dilate, less pumping is required of the heart); also a cerebral vasodilator; decreases release of glutamate (GT); stimulates release of dopamine (DA), acetylcholine (ACh) and serotonin	40 percent experience relief from panic disorder; increases relaxation, energy, exercise tolerance; decreases tender point sensitivity and depression; enhances mental clarity	Diarrhea, low blood pressure, headache	20-40 min	4-8 hrs

DRUG NAME	MARKETED FOR	MODE OF ACTION	EFFECT OF DRUG ON NEUROSOMATIC PATIENTS	POSSIBLE SIDE EFFECTS *	ONSET OF ACTION	DURATION OF ACTION
Gabapentin	Controls epileptic seizures	Enhances releasable pool of GABA in CNS and results in thalamo-cortical excitation; enhances function of thalamic reticular nucleus (RT); may act to reduce centrally mediated pain and enhance slow-wave sleep by inhibiting excitatory neurotrans-mission	Reduces anxiety, depression; increases energy, cognitive clarity, alertness, appetite, stress resistance; relieves headache	Sleepiness, dizziness, fatigue, nausea	30 min	8 hrs
Oxytocin (injection)	Enhances uterine contractions during labor	**Increases peripheral corticotropin-releasing hormone (CRH) secretion; increases NO production	Reduces FMS pain, anxiety, depression; improves cognitive clarity, increases libido	Agitation, high blood pressure, edema	15 min-72 hrs	12-24 hrs
Pyridostigmine	Myasthenia gravis; auto-immune dis-order; muscle weakness	** Peripheral cholinesterase inhibitor (does not cross blood-brain barrier and increases peripheral ACH); may induce adrenal glands to produce more corticoster-oids (such as cortisol) and catecholamines (such as NE and DA); increases secretion of growth hormone (GH)	Reduces muscle weakness, pain; increases energy; improves cognitive clarity	Increased salivation, diarrhea, abdominal cramps, muscle twitching, blurred vision	30 min	4-6 hrs

DRUG NAME	MARKETED FOR	MODE OF ACTION	EFFECT OF DRUG ON NEUROSOMATIC PATIENTS	POSSIBLE SIDE EFFECTS *	ONSET OF ACTION	DURATION OF ACTION
Hydralazine	Generic anti-hypertensive	** Lowers blood pressure by enlarging blood vessels; dilates arteries via NO-type mechanism	Reduces pain, muscle fatigue; increases energy, alertness, memory, cognition, exercise tolerance; enhances restorative sleep	Headache, loss of appetite, nausea vomiting, diarrhea, rapid heartbeat	30-60 min	6-12 hrs
Baclofen	Muscle relaxant; anti-convulsant	Blocks nerve activity in spinal cord (provides supraspinal analgesia; $GABA_B$ agonist) activates $GABA_B$ receptors to hyperpolarize the membrane reducing membrane excitability and the release of neuro-transmitters); inhibits release of CRH and dopamine; stimulates release of GH and insulin-like growth factor-1 (IGF-1)	Provides central pain relief for FMS, low back pain, regional pain syndromes, diffuse pain, headache; reduces anxiety and suppresses panic attacks; increases alertness, energy; reduces MCS and cacosmia	Sedation	30 min	8 hrs
Mexiletine	Antiarrhyth-mic; neuropathic pain (pain, tingling, loss of sense of touch)	** Slows nerve impulses to heart and helps maintain steady rhythm; may act to increase central CRH and inhibit substance P (SP)	Decreases pain, sometimes increases alertness	Nausea, vomiting, diarrhea, constipation, tremors, dizziness, light-headedness, nervousness, poor coordination	30-45 min	6-8 hrs

DRUG NAME	MARKETED FOR	MODE OF ACTION	EFFECT OF DRUG ON NEUROSOMATIC PATIENTS	POSSIBLE SIDE EFFECTS *	ONSET OF ACTION	DURATION OF ACTION
Tacrine	Alzheimer's disease	Centrally acting cholinesterase inhibitor (increases brain ACh); acts as a potassium, calcium, and sodium channel blocker to depolarize cells, producing membrane excitability and release of neurotransmitters; may increase hippocampal NO-synthase activity; prolongs NMDA response, enhancing memory encoding	Increases alertness, energy, feeling of well-being; enhances cognition	Headache, nausea, diarrhea, dizziness, chills, hyperactivity, tingling in hands/feet, respiratory problems	30 min	4-6 hrs
Risperidone	Antipsychotic for treatment of schizophrenia	Serotonin reuptake inhibitor - blocks serotonin destruction at nerve endings); 5-HT$_2$ (serotonin) antagonist (increases glutamate-evoked secretion of NE from the locus ceruleus); could decrease limbic glucocorticoid receptor density and mediate stress response; could enhance midbrain DA release	Increases stage 3 and 4 slow-wave sleep (deep and restorative)	Sedation, movement disorders (rare)	45-60 min	8-12 hrs

DRUG NAME	MARKETED FOR	MODE OF ACTION	EFFECT OF DRUG ON NEUROSOMATIC PATIENTS	POSSIBLE SIDE EFFECTS *	ONSET OF ACTION	DURATION OF ACTION
Pindolol	Hypertension; arrhythmias; anxiety	Beta-adrenergic-blocking agent (beta blockers work by blocking NE and adrenaline from raising heart rate, increasing airflow to the lungs, and dilating blood vessels); a 5-HT$_{1A}$ (serotonin) antagonist (increases GT-evoked secretion of NE from the LC); increases serotonin release in assoc. with antidepressants	General CFS/FMS symptom relief; relief from dyesthesias	Slow heart rate, low blood pressure, may worsen asthma	15 min-7 days	12 hrs
Lamotrigine	Antiepileptic; anticonvulsant	"GABA-mimetic" i.e. mimics effects of GABA); acts in the thalamus to reduce centrally mediated pain by inhibiting excitatory neurotransmissions	Improves alertness; elevates mood	Rash, may increase levels of other antiepileptic drugs	30-45 min	24 hrs
Sumatriptan	Antimigraine	** Constricts blood vessels that are dilated during migraine; 5HT$_{1D}$ (serotonin) agonist (blocks the release of peptides to stop the neurogenic inflammatory response); increases GH and triples neuropeptide Y; may block trigeminal nerve	Decreases pain; eliminates cluster, classic, and common migraines	Chest pain, vertigo, fatigue, worsening of headache, nausea, numbness, a feeling of "strangeness"	15-30 min	16 hrs

74

DRUG NAME	MARKETED FOR	MODE OF ACTION	EFFECT OF DRUG ON NEUROSOMATIC PATIENTS	POSSIBLE SIDE EFFECTS *	ONSET OF ACTION	DURATION OF ACTION
Ranitidine	Antiulcer (stops production of stomach acid)	H2 (histamine) antagonist; may inhibit suppression of IL-1 beta and increase CRH; may increase numbers of natural killer (NK) cells; centrally acting cholinesterase inhibitor (increases brain ACh and central NE)	More energy and alertness; less malaise	Movement disorders, "hyper" feeling	1 hr-1 wk	12-24 hr
Doxepin	Tricyclic anti-depressant, anxiety, chronic pain, panic disorder	Anticholinergic (blocks ACh from occupying cholinergic receptors); reuptake inhibitor for serotonin; strong sedative effect	Improves sleep; decreases pain	Sedation	1 hr	variable
Sertraline	Anti-depres-sant; obses-sive-compul-sive disorder	Prevents movement of serotonin into nerve endings (serotonin stays in spaces around nerve endings where it works)	Improves mood, alertness, energy; decreases pain	Many common side effects but usually not severe	1 hr -6 wks	1-2 days
Bupropion	Antidepres-sant can cause sei-zures	Works chemically to suppress appetite; inhibits NE reuptake	Increases energy and alertness	Dry mouth, diz-ziness, rapid heart-rate, headaches, sweating, intestinal problems, loss of appetite, weight loss, sedation, agitation, blurred vision, trem-ors, sleeplessness	30 min-4 wks	8-24 hrs

DRUG NAME	MARKETED FOR	MODE OF ACTION	EFFECT OF DRUG ON NEUROSOMATIC PATIENTS	POSSIBLE SIDE EFFECTS *	ONSET OF ACTION	DURATION OF ACTION
Nefazodone	Anti-depressant	5-HT$_2$ (serotonin) antagonist (increases GT-evoked NE secretion from the LC); could decrease limbic GR receptor density and mediate stress response; serotonin reuptake inhibitor	Improves mood and sleep	Anxiety, hyperactivity, jerking muscles, if combined with another serotonergic medication ("serotonin syndrome")	2-6 wks	24 hrs
Venlafaxine	Anti-depressant	Serotonin, NE, and DA reuptake inhibitor	May decrease pain and anxiety	Increase in blood pressure, nausea, nervousness, sweating	1-2 wks	24 hrs
Glycine (powder dissolved in juice) or Cycloserine	Antibiotic (Cycloserine used in treatment of tuberculosis)	An inhibitory neurotransmitter in the brainstem and spinal cord; an "obligatory co-agonist" at the NMDA receptor (i.e. unless the glycine site is occupied on the NMDA receptor, the NMDA channel will not open for GT); enhances GT transmission and may increase its release from the PFC	Relieves headaches; increases energy and cognition	Cycloserine may cause depression in antitubercular doses	1 hr	24 hrs

DRUG NAME	MARKETED FOR	MODE OF ACTION	EFFECT OF DRUG ON NEUROSOMATIC PATIENTS	POSSIBLE SIDE EFFECTS *	ONSET OF ACTION	DURATION OF ACTION
Felbamate	Anticonvulsant for seizures; used in mood disorders; used as analgesic	Makes it more difficult for seizures to start or continue; enhances function of $GABA_A$ receptors when GABA neurotransmission is reduced ($GABA_A$ inhibits GT release, slowing energy metabolism); an NMDA receptor antagonist at the glycine co-agonist site	Decreases pain, increases energy	Weight loss, generally well tolerated, side effects vary with dose and other anticonvulsants taken with it, causes aplastic anemia and liver toxicity (rarely); may induce mania (rarely)	30 min	6-8 hrs
Lidocaine (IV injection)	Local anesthetic; analgesic; used for neuropathic pain	** NE, GABA, and choline reuptake inhibitor; stimulates secretion of CRH in hypothalamus; increases rCBF when acting as analgesic; acts at sodium channels to deaden nerve endings when acting as anesthetic; decreases Substance P	Rapidly effective analgesic to reduce FMS pain; when used intranasally, may abort migraines in progress	Nausea, vertigo, numbness, wooziness, seizures, or heart irregularity if given very rapidly	Usually immediately, sometimes takes 24 hours; works better with repeated doses	2 hrs-2 wks

Glossary

Adrenergic: Liberating, activated by or involving adrenaline (also called epinephrine) in the transmission of nerve impulses.

Afferent: Related to nerve fibers that travel from a peripheral site to the brain; proceeding toward a center.

Agonist: A drug that interacts with receptors on cell membranes to initiate a drug response.

Antagonist: A drug that inhibits the action of another drug when both interact at the same receptor site.

Anxiogenic: Producing anxiety.

Anxiolytic: Reducing anxiety.

Attenuate: To reduce the amount, force, or value.

Autonomic Nervous System (ANS): The ANS is responsible for controlling involuntary body functions. It is subdivided into two systems: the sympathetic (SNS), which prepares the body for action (stimulating heart rate, breathing, and sweating, diverting blood to the muscles, and quieting the digestive system), and the parasympathetic (PNS), which dominates during sleep (slowing heart rate and stimulating the digestive system for excretion of waste). The SNS contains chiefly adrenergic fibers (liberating adrenaline, which is also known as epinephrine), as well as noradrenergic fibers (liberating norepinephrine, which is also known as noradrenaline). The PNS contains chiefly cholinergic fibers (liberating acetylcholine).

Beta Blocker: A class of drugs used in the treatment of chest pain caused by insufficient blood flow to the heart, high blood pressure, and cardiac arrhythmias. They may also help reduce the physical symptoms of anxiety and decrease the severity and frequency of migraines. Beta blockers work by binding with beta-receptors found in the heart, as well as the lungs, blood vessels, and other tissues. The neurotransmitters epinephrine (adrenaline) and norepinephrine bind with the beta-receptors to increase the heart beat, increase airflow to the lungs and dilate blood vessels. Beta blocker drugs reverse the effect of these neurotransmitters, slowing the heart rate and reducing the force of the heart's contractions. Elsewhere in the body, beta blockers can reduce muscle tremor associated with anxiety and calm an overactive thyroid gland.

Blood-Brain Barrier: A network of uniquely structured blood vessels, these capillaries are nearly impermeable to many toxic chemicals carried by the blood. Oxygen, water, carbon dioxide, glucose, the essential amino acids from food, and a few other substances with specific characteristics are allowed to pass through the barrier. Caffeine, nicotine, and alcohol are among these, accounting for their rapid and profound effect on mood. Certain foods, too, can influence moods by virtue of their amino acids, which can pass through the barrier. It helps to drink milk before bed, for instance, because the amino acid tryptophan enters the brain where it is converted to serotonin, which is involved in sleep.

Cacosmia: An individual's perception of an odor, which is inapparent to others and produces feelings of illness.

Calcium Channel Blockers: A class of drugs used in the treatment of chest pain caused by insufficient blood flow to the heart, high blood pressure, and cardiac arrhythmias. Calcium channel blockers work by preventing the movement of calcium across the membrane lining muscle cells, interfering with the process of contraction. As the muscles relax and dilate, blood circulation through the heart muscle is increased, and blood flow is increased throughout the tissues, requiring less pumping action by the heart. These drugs also slow the transmission of nerve impulses through the heart muscle, correcting certain kinds of arrhythmias.

Cerebrospinal Fluid (CSF): A watery fluid produced by specialized structures within the brain called choroid plexuses. The CSF circulates between the ventricles (cavities) within the brain and continuously washes over the brain and spinal cord to cushion them from injury.

Cholinergic: Liberating, activated by, or involving acetylcholine in the transmission of nerve impulses.

Cholinesterase Inhibitor: A substance that inhibits the enzyme cholinesterase in the breakdown of acetylcholine, effectively increasing brain levels of acetylcholine.

Deafferentation: The suppression or loss of afferent nerve impulses traveling to the brain from a peripheral site.

Denervation Hypersensitivity: If a neurotransmitter is not secreted in sufficient quantity, its receptors increase in number and/or sensitivity in an attempt to most effectively utilize the available neurotransmitter.

Depolarized: A nerve cell that has an increased membrane potential due to decreased potassium (K) conductance (i.e., potassium ions are confined to intracellular space); neuronal excitability is increased; opposite of hyperpolarized.

Desensitization: Tolerance to once-effective drugs that appears to be related to reduced response to receptor stimulation. This can occur in two forms: "uncoupling," a loss of signal function, and "downregulation," a loss of receptor number. In the first case, a receptor is "phosphorylated," which results in increasing its affinity for an inhibitor substance, which then uncouples it from its stimulatory substance. In the second case, a receptor can be more rapidly degraded or less rapidly manufactured, both of which can result in downregulation.

Dystonia: Abnormal tone usually occurring in muscles.

Efferent: Related to nerve fibers that travel from the brain to peripheral sites within the body; directed away from a center.

Endothelium: A single cell layer that lines all internal body cavities. Endothelial cells in the brain secrete nitric oxide (NO), essential in the process of long-term-potentiation (LTP), involved in memory encoding.

-ergic: A suffix denoting an agent that causes the release of a neurotransmitter from a nerve terminal, as in gabaergic, serotonergic, glutamatergic, dopaminergic, or histaminergic.

Ganglion: A collection of nerve cell bodies located outside the brain and spinal cord; autonomic ganglia refer to ganglia within the sympathetic and parasympathetic nervous systems (SNS and PNS).

Glucocorticoid: A corticoid (such as cortisol) that increases liver glycogen and blood sugar by increasing the production of glucose from the liver.

Heteromodal Association Areas: Regions of the cerebral cortex that do not receive sensory information directly, but coordinate complex preprocessed data from more than one sensory sphere. They can integrate smell, taste, and sight; sensory and motor experiences; and information from both the outside world and the internal milieu.

Hyperperfusion: Increased cerebral blood flow.

Hypoperfusion: Reduced cerebral blood flow.

Hyperpolarized: A nerve cell that has a decreased membrane potential due to increased potassium (K) conductance (i.e., the movement of potassium ions from intracellular to extracellular space); neuronal excitability is decreased; opposite of depolarized.

Neocortex: the dorsal (posterior) region of the cortex; the most recently developed part of the brain that is unique to mammals.

Noradrenergic: Liberating, activated by, or involving norepinephrine (also called noradrenaline) in the transmission of nerve impulses.

Nitric Oxide (NO) synthase: The enzyme that acts on arginine to manufacture NO.

Postganglionic: Situated behind or distal to (farthest from) a ganglion.

Preganglionic: Situated before or proximal to a ganglion (nearest to the center).

rCBF: An abbreviation for "regional cerebral blood flow."

Reuptake Inhibitor: A drug that blocks the reuptake (a sort of reabsorption) of a neurotransmitter at nerve endings, allowing it to exert a longer lasting effect and compensate for deficient levels; most are termed "selective," meaning that they do not disrupt the action of other neurotransmitters; as in selective serotonin reuptake inhibitors (SRIs).

Secretagogue: A substance that stimulates the secretion of another substance.

Ventricles: A system of four communication cavities within the brain, filled with cerebrospinal fluid and linked by ducts, allowing the fluid to circulate through them. The ventricles contain specialized structures called choroid plexuses, which secrete the cerebrospinal fluid.

References

Bennett, Robert. (1995). Patient Conference, Sacramento, CA, January, as reported by *Fibromyalgia Network*, 30, July 1995, p. 3.

Bennett, Robert and Russell, I. Jon. (1993). From a presentation by I. Jon Russell at the American College of Rheumatology conference in San Antonio, TX, November 7-11, as reported by *Fibromyalgia Network*, 25, April 1994, p. 5.

Goldstein, Jay A. (1993). *Chronic Fatigue Syndromes: The Limbic Hypothesis*. Binghamton, NY: The Haworth Medical Press, Inc.

Goldstein, Jay A. (1996). *Betrayal By the Brain: The Neurological Basis of Chronic Fatigue Syndrome, Fibromyalgia Syndrome, and Related Neural Network Disorders*. Binghamton, NY: The Haworth Medical Press, Inc.

Poole, Robert M., ed., (1986). *The Incredible Machine*. Washington, DC: National Geographic Society.

Index

Page numbers followed by the letter "t" indicate tables.

T - #0606 - 101024 - C0 - 212/152/5 - PB - 9780789001191 - Gloss Lamination